A Practical Guide To Transcranial Doppler Examinations

Mira L. Katz, Ph.D., MPH, RVT

and

Andrei V. Alexandrov, M.D., RVT

Published by Summer Publishing

Summer Publishing, LLC
4572 Christensen Circle
Littleton, CO 80123
USA

303-734-1789
fax- 1-866-519-0674
email address: Info@summerpublishing.com
website: www.summerpublishing.com

Cover design by Pam McKinnie, Concepts Unlimited

Cover illustrations and images courtesy of:
Nicolet Vascular, Madison, WI
Philips Ultrasound, Bothell, WA
Spencer Technologies, Seattle, WA

ISBN 978-0-9720653-1-3

Preface

This guide is an introduction to the techniques and the interpretation of transcranial Doppler (TCD) and transcranial color Doppler imaging (TCDI) examinations. It is intentionally written at an introductory level. Emphasis is placed on intracranial anatomy, examination techniques, and the interpretation of the TCD data. Performing a technically excellent TCD examination requires full understanding of the involved basic sciences. It is beyond the scope of this guide, however, to review all topics associated with performing TCD examinations. Although in-depth information regarding cerebrovascular physiology, patho-physiology, or the physical principles associated with diagnostic Doppler ultrasound are not included, these important topics are referenced throughout this guide.

In both chapters dedicated to technique, replication of common issues (locating the ultrasound window, patient positioning, etc.) associated with the transcranial Doppler and the transcranial color Doppler imaging examination can be found. This was intentionally done so that each chapter would individually contain all the important information needed to perform a TCD or TCDI examination.

It is our hope that this guide is useful to the new user by providing a basic and detailed presentation on how to perform a TCD or a TCDI examination and how to interpret the results.

Mira L. Katz, Ph.D., M.P.H., R.V.T.
Andrei V. Alexandrov, M.D., R.V.T.

CONTENTS

Preface

Chapter 1. Introduction....1

Chapter 2. Anatomy For TCD Examinations....9

Chapter 3. Transcranial Doppler Technique....25

Chapter 4. Transcranial Color Doppler Imaging....49

Chapter 5. Normal Values & Physiologic Variables....79

Chapter 6. Clinical Applications....91

Chapter 7. Case Examples.... 127

Chapter 8. TCD Report Forms & Protocol....135

Comprehensive Examination....143

Answers: Cases & Comprehensive Examination....153

Index 157

Chapter 1
Introduction

Stroke is the third leading cause of death in the United States. Approximately 160,000 of the 750,000 strokes that occur each year result in death.[1] Stroke is also a leading cause of adult disability. Although the risk of stroke dramatically increases with age, the incidence of pediatric stroke is also on the rise. In addition, the direct (hospital, physician, rehabilitation, etc.) and indirect (lost productivity, etc.) costs associated with stroke tally more than $30 billion per year in the United States.[1]

The prevention of stroke has been the focus for the progress made in the ultrasound evaluation of cerebrovascular disease during the past twenty years. Development of an ultrasound method to interrogate the intracranial arterial system, however, lagged behind the evaluation of the extracranial arterial system because of the attention focused on surgically correctable lesions of the carotid bifurcation, and the difficulty penetrating the skull with ultrasound. Recent technical advancements permit the ultrasonic evaluation of the intracranial arterial system by using transcranial Doppler (TCD).[2] Initially, the operator may find it difficult to perform a non-imaging TCD examination due to "blind" placement of the Doppler sample volume. Proper examination technique, intracranial arterial identification criteria, and experience will minimize this concern. The operator must be aware that the Doppler spectral waveforms obtained during a TCD examination are based on hemodynamics, and that the waveforms obtained do not provide anatomic information.

It is critical to understand that TCD measures the velocity of the blood and does not measure cerebral blood flow. Increases in intracranial arterial velocity may be due but not limited to: increased volume flow without a lumen diameter change, a decrease in lumen diameter (stenosis) without a change in volume flow, or by a combination of an increase in volume flow and a decrease in lumen diameter.

Technical advancements during the past few years have lead to the development of multi-gated TCD as well as M (motion)-mode power Doppler and transcranial color Doppler imaging (TCDI). M-mode color TCD may assist the operator in locating the best TCD windows, in accurately identifying the intracranial arteries, in the identification of emboli, and in a rapid assessment of directionality changes during monitoring.[3,4] TCDI is an advancement of intracranial ultrasound techniques since it combines the hemodynamic information with anatomic landmarks, enabling the accurate identification of the intracranial arteries. TCDI may also provide important ancillary anatomic information.[5,6]

This chapter describes: 1) the role of the TCD operator, 2) the importance of performing carotid duplex imaging prior to the TCD examination, and 3) the clinical areas which may benefit by the addition of an ultrasound evaluation of the intracranial vasculature.

Operator

The most critical factor in performing accurate TCD examinations is the operator. It is overly optimistic to suggest that all users of TCD equipment will have the same level of diagnostic ability. TCD is not a simple technique. It's diagnostic acumen is dependent upon the skill and experience of the operator and of the interpreter. While experience is important with any ultrasound technology, the importance of proper technique and understanding the principles of Doppler ultrasound physics, cerebrovascular anatomy and physiology, and the pathophysiology of the various related disease processes cannot be overstated.

Even though transcranial Doppler and transcranial color Doppler imaging may share many of the basic principles that apply to the ultrasound evaluation of the cervical carotid arteries, TCD elevates the operator to a new integrative plateau. Alert thinking and a willingness to prevail over a diagnostic enigma are important characteristics for the operator. To perform a good quality examination and to make an accurate interpretation, the operator must consolidate the TCD data with: 1) the status of the patient's extracranial arteries, 2) the patient's individual physiologic parameters (i.e. age, hematocrit, etc.), 3) the patient's neurological signs and symptoms, and 4) the understanding of the limitations of the technique.

The operator must exercise complete concentration when performing a TCD examination. The value of the hemodynamic information obtained during a TCD examination directly correlates to its quality. To perform accurate TCD examinations, the operator must have patience and uninterrupted examination time. Depending on the difficulty of the examination, i.e. locating the TCD windows, a complete TCD examination may take 30 to 60 minutes.

It is also important that the operator have the appropriate education and training prior to performing and interpreting TCD examinations. Certification of technologists, sonographers, and physicians, and the accreditation of the department responsible for the TCD evaluations are critical steps in ensuring uniform and acceptable quality care and patient safety.[7-9]

Another critical factor when performing TCD examinations is the operator's communication skills. This is important when the operator explains the test to patients, and is also critical when trying to convey the results of the examination to other healthcare professionals.

Carotid Duplex Imaging

The accurate interpretation of a patient's TCD examination may be very difficult without knowledge of the location and the extent of atherosclerotic disease present in the extracranial vasculature. Duplex imaging is currently used to assess the cervical portion of the cerebrovascular system (Figure 1-1). Duplex imaging provides valuable information about the amount of disease present (percent diameter reduction), the length of the plaque, and the localized hemodynamic effects of the atherosclerotic plaque (Figure 1-2). Carotid and vertebral duplex imaging techniques, interpretation criteria, and diagnostic capabilities are established.[10-28] There have been multiple diagnostic criteria (peak systolic velocity, end diastolic velocity, internal carotid artery (ICA)/common carotid artery (CCA) ratios) for varying degrees of narrowing of the proximal ICA suggested by various investigators. The most important recommendation is that each institution establishes its own diagnostic criteria by comparing carotid duplex imaging with conventional arteriography or magnetic resonance arteriography.[29] Adding color and power Doppler to duplex imaging may be helpful in: the rapid identification of an area of stenosis, the accurate placement of the sample volume in the area of the stenosis, readily identifying normal and tortuous vessels (Figure 1-3), in the identification of the origin of the vertebral arteries, and determining arterial occlusion versus a high grade stenosis. It is the identification of color patterns, in conjunction with the conventional carotid duplex imaging velocity criteria that may improve the overall accuracy of the technique.

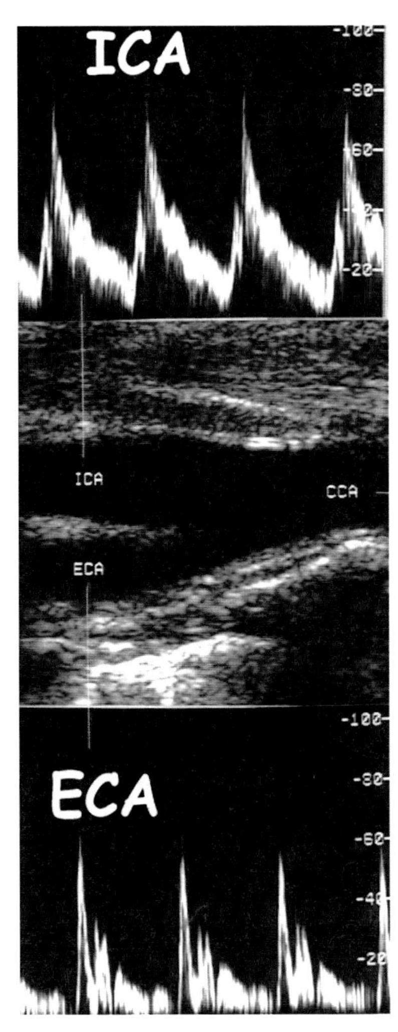

Figure 1-1. An image of a normal common carotid artery (CCA) bifurcation and the spectral Doppler waveforms obtained from the internal carotid artery (ICA) and the external carotid artery (ECA).

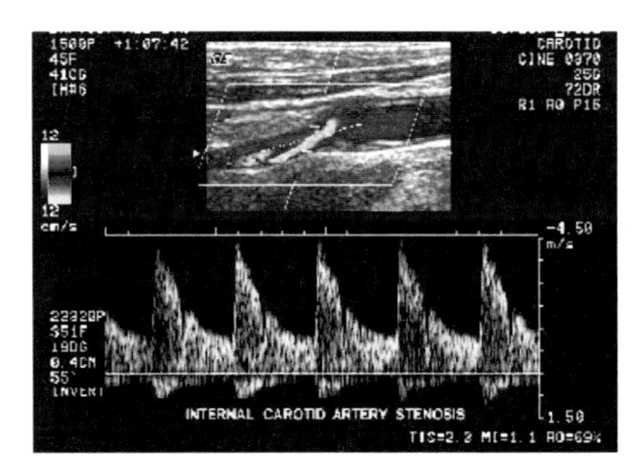

Figure 1-2. A stenosis of the internal carotid artery. There is an increase in the peak systolic velocity. [Courtesy of GE Ultrasound Company]

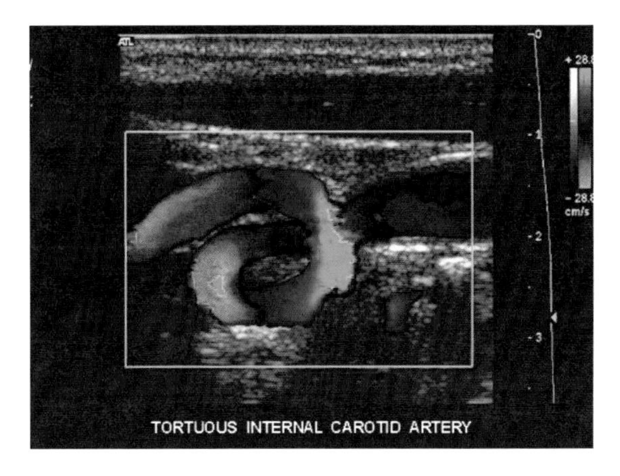

Figure 1-3. Color Doppler imaging of a tortuous internal carotid artery. [Courtesy of Philips Ultrasound Company]

Duplex imaging may also provide information about the morphological characteristics of the plaque and plaque structure which may prove to be important in its association with patient symptoms.[30-36] Carotid duplex imaging is also being used to evaluate the status of the arteries pre and post stent placement.[36-38] Carotid ultrasound documents the stent location, patency and thrombosis, and the evaluation of the proximal and distal arteries (Figure 1-4). Additionally, carotid duplex imaging is being used to measure the intima-media thickness (IMT) of the common carotid artery. Measurement of IMT may predict patients who are at risk for stroke and myocardial infarction.[39,40] Standardization of instrument controls and diagnostic criteria are needed, however, prior to determining the definitive role of carotid duplex imaging in these areas.

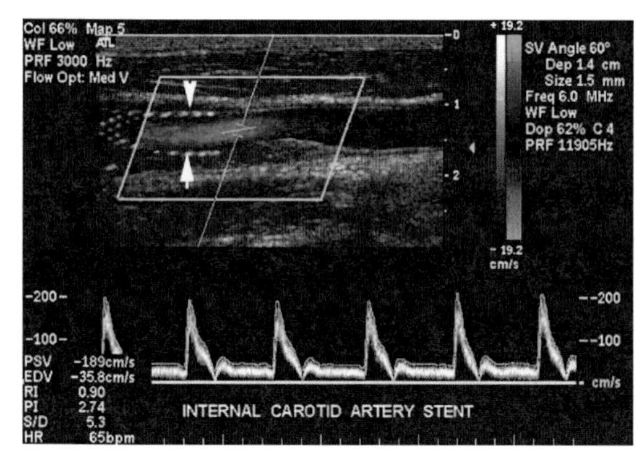

Figure 1-4. A stent visualized in the ICA. [Courtesy of Philips Ultrasound Company]

When performing TCD and TCDI examinations it is important to know the status of the extracranial arteries because extensive extracranial disease may cause changes in the velocity and/or direction of blood flow in a patient's intracranial arterial system. Transcranial Doppler gives us the opportunity to evaluate the hemodynamic effects of extracranial occlusive disease on intracranial blood flow.

Additionally, carotid duplex imaging can determine the level of the common carotid bifurcation and if any disease is present in the common carotid artery. This is extremely important if the operator is performing common carotid artery (CCA) compression in conjunction with the TCD examination. ***Common carotid artery compressions are not routinely performed during TCD examinations, and should be performed only by experienced personnel and only if the patient has a disease free CCA.*** This information is easily obtained by carotid duplex imaging.

Although atherosclerotic disease usually occurs in the area of the CCA bifurcation, it often can be found along the walls of the CCA. Compression of a diseased CCA might dislodge friable atheromatous debris, causing a cerebral embolus. Thromboembolic complications have been reported as a result of performing CCA compression during a TCD examination.[41] The visualization of atherosclerotic disease in the CCA in many patients prompts this warning about common carotid artery compression.

Clinical Applications

The transcranial Doppler technique was introduced as a method to detect cerebral arterial vasospasm following subarachnoid hemorrhage.[42,43] During the past 20 years, the list of clinical applications for TCD has grown, and the addition of new areas of research will permit better understanding of intracranial cerebrovascular hemodynamics.[44]

Currently, transcranial Doppler's role is being used or investigated for the following clinical applications:

- Diagnosis of intracranial vascular disease
- Monitoring vasospasm in subarachnoid hemorrhage
- Screening of children with sickle cell disease
- Assessment of intracranial collateral pathways
- Evaluation of the hemodynamic effects of extracranial occlusive disease on intracranial blood flow
- Intraoperative monitoring

- Detection of cerebral emboli
- Monitoring evolution of cerebral circulatory arrest
- Documentation of subclavian steal
- Evaluation of the vertebrobasilar system
- Detection of feeders ofarteriovenous malformations (AVMs)
- Monitoring anticoagulation regimens or thrombolytic therapy
- Monitoring during neuroradiologic interventions
- Testing of functional reserve
- Monitoring after head trauma

Although the Doppler evaluation and the color Doppler imaging examination of the intracranial arteries are still under development, TCD will evolve further, and our understanding of its clinical usefulness will become more apparent in the coming years.

References

1. National Stroke Association. http://www.stroke.org Accessed 2002.
2. Aaslid R, Markwalder T-M, Nornes H. Noninvasive transcranial Doppler ultrasound recording of flow velocity in basal cerebral arteries. J Neurosurg 1982;57:769-774.
3. Moehring MA, Spencer MP. Power M-mode Doppler (PMD) for observing cerebral blood flow and tracking emboli. Ultrasound Med Biol 2002;28:49-57.
4. Alexandrov AV, Demchuk AM, Burgin WS. Insonation method and diagnostic flow signatures for transcranial power motion (M-mode) Doppler. J Neuroimaging 2002;12:236-244.
5. Schoning M, Buchholz R, Walter J. Comparative study of transcranial color duplex sonography and transcranial Doppler sonography in adults. J Neurosurg 1993;78:776-784.
6. Becker G, Seufert J, Bogdahn U, et al. Degeneration of substantia nigra in chronic Parkinson's disease visualized by transcranial color-coded real-time sonography. Neurology 1995;45:182-184.
7. American Registry of Diagnostic Medical Sonographers (ARDMS). http://www.ardms.org
8. Intersocietal Commission for the Accreditation of Vascular Laboratories (ICAVL). http://www.icavl.org
9. American Institute of Ultrasound in Medicine (AIUM). http://www.aium.org
10. Primozich JF. Extracranial Arterial Disease. In: Duplex Scanning In Vascular Disorders. 3rd Edition, DE Strandness, Jr. (ed), Philadelphia, Lippincott, Williams & Wilkins, 2002.
11. Polak JF. Carotid Ultrasound. Radiol Clin North Am 2001;39:569-589.
12. Polak JF. Color flow imaging of the carotid arteries. In: Tegler CH, Babikian VL, Gomez CR (eds): Neurosonology. St. Louis: Mosby-Year Book, Chapter 9, 1996:68-82.

13. Huston J, James EM, Brown RD et al. Redefined duplex ultrasonographic criteria for diagnosis of carotid artery stenosis. Mayo Clin Proc 2000; 75:1133-1140.

14. Moneta GL, Edwards JM, Chitwood RW et al. Correlation of North America Symptomatic Carotid Endarterectomy Trial (NASCET) angiographic definition of 70-99% internal carotid artery stenosis with duplex scanning. J Vasc Surg 1993; 17:152-159.

15. Moneta GL, Edwards JM, Papanicolaou G et al. Screening for asymptomatic carotid internal carotid artery stenosis: duplex criteria for discriminating 60-99% stenosis. J Vasc Surg 1995;21:989-994.

16. Hood DB, Mattos MA, Mansour A, et al. Prospective evaluation of new duplex criteria to identify a 70% internal carotid stenosis. J Vasc Surg 1996; 23:254-262.

17. Lee VS, Hertzberg BS, Kliewer MA, Carroll BA. Assessment of stenosis: implications of variability of Doppler measurements in normal-appearing carotid arteries. Radiology 1999; 212:493-498.

18. Carpenter JP, Lexa FJ, Davis JT. Determination of duplex Doppler ultrasound criteria appropriate to the North American Symptomatic Carotid Endarterectomy Trial. Stroke 1996; 27:695-699.

19. Carpenter JP, Lexa FJ, Davis JT. Determination of sixty percent or greater carotid artery stenosis by duplex Doppler ultrasonography. J Vasc Surg 1995; 22:697-705.

20. Fillinger MF, Baker RJ, Zwolak RM et al. Carotid duplex criteria for a 60% or greater angiographic stenosis: variation according to equipment. J Vasc Surg. 1996;24:856-864.

21. Nehler MR, Moneta GL, Lee RW et al. Improving selection of patients with less than 60% asymptomatic internal carotid artery stenosis for follow-up of carotid artery duplex scanning. J Vasc Surg 1996;23:580-587.

22. Grant EG, Duerinckx AJ, ElSaden S, et al. Doppler sonographic parameters for detection of carotid stenosis: is there an optimum method for their selection? AJR 1999;172:1123-1129.

23. Grant EG, Duerinckx AJ, ElSaden SM, et al. Ability to use duplex US to quantify internal carotid arterial stenoses: fact or fiction? Radiology 2000;214:247-252.

24. Fujitani RM, Mills JL, Wang LM, Taylor SM. The effect of unilateral internal carotid artery occlusion upon contralateral duplex study: criteria for accurate interpretation. J Vasc Surg 1992;16:459-468.

25. Busuttil SJ, Franklin DP, Youkey JR, Elmore JR. Carotid duplex overestimation of stenosis due to severe contralateral disease. Am J Surg 1996;172:144-148.

26. Bluth EI, Merritt CR, Sullivan MA, et al. Usefulness of duplex ultrasound in evaluating vertebral arteries. J Ultrasound Med 1989;8:229-235.

27. Trattnig S, Hubsch P, Schuster H, Polzleitner D. Color-coded Doppler imaging of normal vertebral arteries. Stroke 1990;21:1222-1225.

28. Bartels E. Vertebral sonography. In: Tegler CH, Babikian VL, Gomez CR (eds): Neurosonology. St. Louis: Mosby-Year Book; Chapter 10, 1996:83-100.

29. Kuntz KM, Polak JF, Whittemore AD, et al. Duplex ultrasound criteria for the identification of carotid stenosis should be laboratory specific. Stroke 1997; 28:597-602.

30. Tegos TJ, Kalomiris KJ, Sabetai MM, et al. Significance of sonographic tissue and surface characteristics of carotid plaques. AJNR 2001;22:1605-1612.

31. Tegos TJ, Stavropoulos P, Sabetai MM, et al. Determinants of carotid plaque instability: echoicity versus heterogeneity. Eur J Vasc Endovasc Surg 2001;22:22-3.

32. Reilly LM, Lusby RJ, Hughes L, et al. Carotid plaque histology using real-time ultrasonography: clinical and therapeutic implications. Am J Surg 1983;146:188-193.

33. Comerota AJ, Katz ML, White JV, Grosh JD. The preoperative diagnosis of the ulcerated carotid atheroma. J Vasc Surg 1990;11:505-510.

34. Sitzer M, Muller W, Rademacher J et. al. Color-flow Doppler-assisted duplex imaging fails to detect ulceration in high-grade internal carotid artery stenosis. J Vasc Surg 1996;23:461-465.

35. Arnold JAC, Modaresi KB, Thomas N, et al. Carotid plaque characterization by duplex scanning: observer error may undermine current clinical trials. Stroke 1999;30:61-65.

36. AbuRahma AF, Covelli MA, Robinson PA, Holt SM. The role of carotid duplex ultrasound in evaluating plaque morphology: potential use in selecting patients for carotid stenting. J Endovasc Surg 1999;6:59-65.

37. Chakhtoura EY, Hobson RW, Goldstein J, et al. In-stent restenosis after carotid angioplasty-stenting: incidence and management. J Vasc Surg 2001;33:220-226.

38. Robbin ML, Lockhart ME, Weber TM et al. Carotid artery stents: early and intermediate follow-up with Doppler US. Radiology 1997;205:749-756.

39. O'Leary DH, Polak JF, Kronmal RA et al. Carotid-artery intima and media thickness as a risk factor for myocardial infarction and stroke in older adults. N Engl J Med 1999;340:14-22.

40. Chambless LE, Folsom AR, Clegg LX et al. Carotid wall thickness is predictive of incident clinical stroke: the Atherosclerosis Risk in Communities (ARIC) Study. Am J Epidemiol 2000;151:478-487.

41. Khaffaf N, Karnik R, Winkler W-B, et al. Embolic stroke by compression maneuver during transcranial Doppler sonography. Stroke 1994;25:1056-1057.

42. Aaslid R, Huber P, Nornes H. Evaluation of cerebrovascular spasm with transcranial Doppler ultrasound. J Neurosurg 1984;60:37-41.

43. Lindegaard KF, Nornes H, Bakke SJ, Sorteberg W, Nakstad P. Cerebral vasospasm after subarachnoid haemorrhage investigated by means of transcranial Doppler ultrasound. Acta Neurochir(Wien) 1988;42 Suppl:P81-84.

44. Babikian VL, Feldmann E, Wechsler LR, et al. Transcranial Doppler ultrasonography: Year 2000 update. J Neuroimaging 2000;10:101-115.

Additional Readings

Kremkau FW. Doppler Ultrasound: Principles and Instruments. 6th ed. Philadelphia: WB Saunders, 2002.

Zagzebski JA. Essentials of ultrasound physics. St. Louis: Mosby, 1997.

Chapter 2
Anatomy For TCD Examinations

An anterior (carotid) and a posterior (vertebral) circulation supply blood to the brain. Familiarity with the anatomy of the major intracranial vessels (Figure 2-1) is requisite to performing accurate transcranial Doppler (TCD) and transcranial color Doppler imaging examinations.

This chapter describes: 1) the anterior and posterior cerebrovascular systems, 2) common anatomic variations of these systems, and 3) interconnections between these systems.

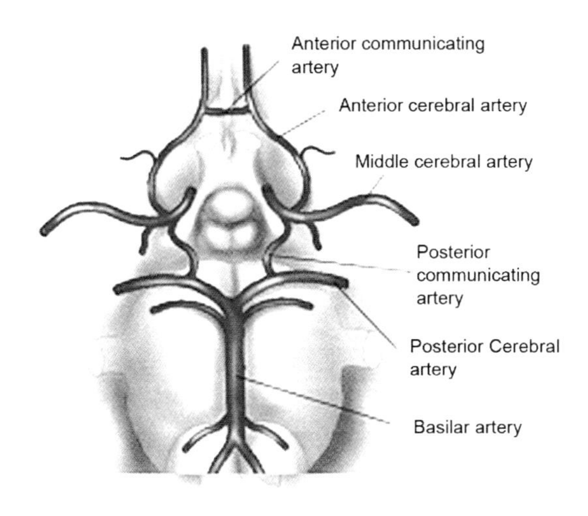

Figure 2-1. The circle of Willis and the vertebrobasilar arterial system. [From:Katz ML. Intracranial Cerebrovascular Evaluation. In: Textbook of Diagnostic Ultrasonography. Mosby, St. Louis, 2001]

Skull and Brain[1-7]

During a successful TCD examination, ultrasound waves penetrate selected areas of the skull. The following is a brief description of TCD landmarks.

The skull consists of twenty-one bones that are fused, and one moveable bone, the mandible. The majority of the cranial bones consist of three layers. The middle layer, the diplöe, separates the internal and external laminae. The diplöe is a layer of cancellous bone and plays an important role in the attenuation and scattering of ultrasound waves. The inner and outer layers are compact ivory bone and cause refraction of the ultrasound waves.

There is substantial variability in the thickness of the bone between individuals. Grolimund described the influence of skull thickness on a focused ultrasound beam.[4] He found that the mean loss of power transversing the skull was approximately 80%. This loss of power during insonation through the skull is one of the major technical limitations of TCD examinations.

The lateral surface of the skull is the temporal bone, which forms most of the skull's lower lateral section. The zygomatic bone, the bony prominence of the cheek, projects a frontal process upward and a temporal process horizontally and backwards towards the temporal bone. The temporal process of the zygomatic bone and the zygomatic process of the temporal bone form the zygomatic arch. The transtemporal TCD approach is through the squamous portion of the temporal bone superior to the zygomatic arch. This area of the temporal bone is the thinnest part of the skull, making it technically possible for ultrasound insonation of the intracranial arteries in the majority of adults. The transtemporal window is generally the most informative approach of the TCD examination, and is used to evaluate the terminal internal carotid artery, the middle cerebral artery, the anterior cerebral artery, the posterior cerebral artery, and the anterior and posterior communicating arteries.

Anteriorly, the maxilla and the ethmoid bones form most of the inferior and medial borders of the orbit. The lateral border is formed by the zygomatic bone and the greater wing of the sphenoid bone. The frontal bone and the lesser wing of the sphenoid bone form the roof of the orbit. Recently, frontal bone windows were described to evaluate A2 segments of the anterior cerebral arteries, however insonation failures are more common with this approach than with transtemporal windows.[7]

The supraorbital foramen, through which the supraorbital artery runs, is located on the supraorbital margin of the frontal bone. The optic canals are round ostia (openings) at the back of the orbits that lie in the lesser wing of the sphenoid bone. During the transorbital approach of a TCD examination, the ophthalmic artery and the internal carotid artery siphon are evaluated by using the ostia at the back of the orbits.

The occipital bone is the prominent posterior aspect of the skull and forms part of its base. The large oval opening in this bone is the foramen magnum. The suboccipital approach of a TCD examination uses this ostium to evaluate the intracranial vertebral arteries and the basilar artery.

The petrous portion of the temporal bone, incorporating the jugular foramen and the carotid canal, forms the posterior part of the skull lateral to the occipital bone. The petrous apex is the portion of the temporal bone just anterior to the ear. It presents the anterior or internal orifice of the carotid canal and forms the posterolateral boundary of the foramen lacerum. During a TCD examination, the carotid canal is used for the submandibular approach allowing ultrasonic access to the retromandibular segment of the internal carotid artery.

The brain is housed within the cranial cavity and is covered by three membranes called meninges. The outermost layer, the dura mater (pachymenix), is a dense fibrous sheath overlying the thin subdural space between the dura mater and the middle layer, the arachnoid mater. The arachnoid mater is a thin, delicate, spider web-like membrane. It is separated from the inner layer, the pia mater, by the subarachnoid space. The subarachnoid space contains the cerebrospinal fluid and the large blood vessels of the brain. The innermost layer, the pia mater, is a thin vascular membrane that closely adheres to the brain. It carries blood vessels that supply the neural tissue. The arachnoid and the pia mater are collectively referred to as the leptomeninges.

The brain is formed by the cerebrum (two large paired cerebral hemispheres and the diencephalon), the cerebellum, and the brainstem. The right and left hemispheres of the cerebrum constitute the largest part of the brain. They are separated by the longitudinal cerebral fissure and are connected at the bottom by a mass of white matter, the corpus callosum. The falx cerebri is a small fold of the dura mater that is located between the hemispheres. A second fold of dura mater, called the tentorium cerebelli, separates the cerebral hemispheres from the cerebellum. This structure is rigid and splits intracranial space into supra- and infratentorial portions.

Each hemisphere is divided into five lobes; the frontal, temporal, occipital, parietal, and insular. The Sylvian fissure, also called the lateral sulcus, separates the temporal lobe from the parietal and frontal lobes. The blood supply to the majority of the lateral surface of the cerebral hemispheres is by the middle cerebral arteries, while the anterior cerebral and posterior cerebral arteries supply most of the medial and inferior surfaces.

The cerebellum lies immediately below the posterior portion of the cerebral hemispheres. It consists of paired laterally and posteriorly protruding cerebellar hemispheres and a smaller continuous midline portion, the vermis. The cerebellum is supplied by the paired cerebellar arteries; the posterior inferior cerebellar (PICA), anterior inferior cerebellar (AICA), and superior cerebellar arteries (SCA), which are branches of the vertebrobasilar system.

The brainstem consists of the medulla oblongata (myelencephalon), the pons or metencephalon, and the midbrain or mesencephalon. Each half of the midbrain is called a cerebral peduncle and consists of heavy fiber bundles. The branches of the vertebrobasilar system, the posterior cerebral arteries, and the posterior communicating arteries supply the brainstem.

CEREBRAL CIRCULATION

Aortic Arch[8-12]

The ascending aorta originates from the left ventricle of the heart. The transverse aortic arch lies in the superior mediastinum and is formed as the aorta ascends and curves posteroinferiorly from right to left, above the left mainstem bronchus. It descends to the left of the trachea and esophagus. Three main arteries arise from the superior convexity of the arch in its normal configuration. The brachiocephalic trunk (innominate artery) is the first branch, the left common carotid artery the second, and the left subclavian artery the third branch in approximately 70% of cases.

The brachiocephalic trunk divides into the right common carotid and the right subclavian artery, which gives rise to the right vertebral. The left common carotid artery originates slightly to the left of the innominate artery, followed by the left subclavian, which likewise gives rise to the left vertebral artery.

Anatomic variants of the major arch vessels occur frequently. The most common variant (approximately 10%) is the left common carotid artery forming a common origin with or originating directly from the innominate artery. Less frequently the left vertebral artery arises directly from the arch, the right subclavian artery originates from the arch distal to the left subclavian artery, the right common carotid artery originates directly from the arch, and a left innominate artery may exist from which the left common carotid and left subclavian originate.

ANTERIOR CIRCULATION

Common Carotid Artery[13]

Each common carotid artery (CCA) ascends through the superior mediastinum anterolaterally in the neck and lies medial to the jugular vein. The left common carotid is usually longer than the right, because it originates from the aortic arch. In the neck, the carotid artery, jugular vein, and vagus nerve are enclosed in connective tissue called the carotid sheath. The vagus nerve lies between and dorsal to the artery and vein. The CCA usually does not have branches, but occasionally the superior thyroid artery originates from it. The common carotid artery's termination is the carotid bifurcation, which is the origin of the external carotid artery (ECA) and the internal carotid artery (ICA) (Figure 2-2). The CCA bifurcates in the vicinity of the superior border of the thyroid cartilage (approximately C4) in 70% of the cases, and the level of the CCA

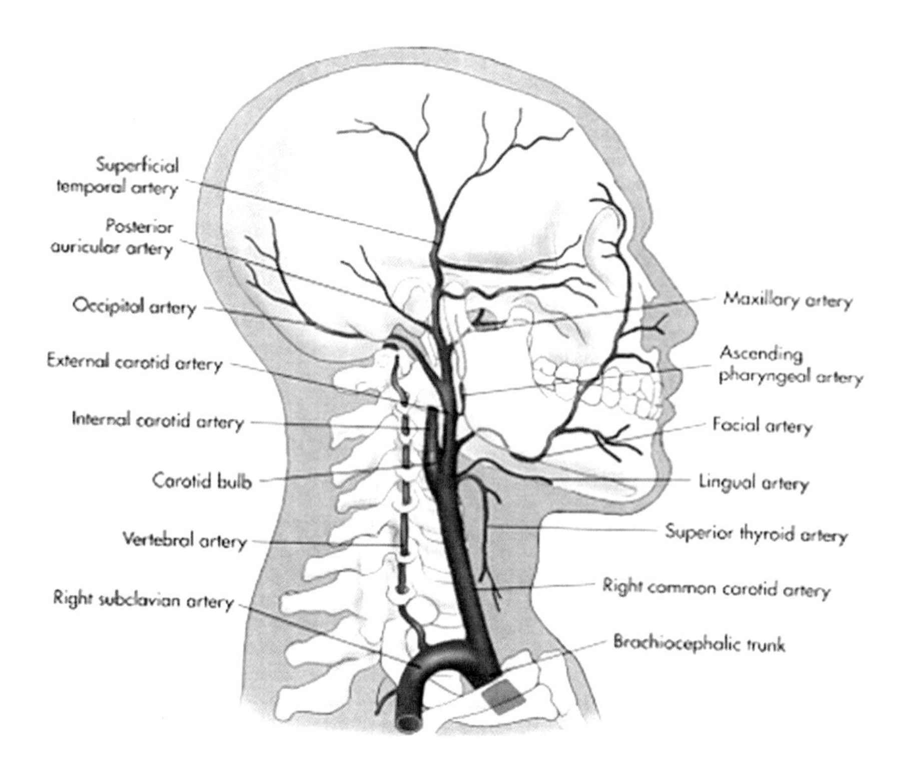

Figure 2-2. The common carotid artery bifurcation is the origin of the internal and external carotid arteries. [From: Katz ML. Extracranial Cerebrovascular Evaluation. In: Textbook of Diagnostic Ultrasonography. Mosby, St. Louis, 2001]

bifurcations may be asymmetrical. The CCA bifurcation has been described as low as T2 and as high as C1.

External Carotid Artery[14,15]

The external carotid artery originates at the mid-cervical level and is usually the smaller of the two terminal branches of the CCA. Initially it lies anteromedial to the internal carotid artery, but as the ECA ascends it courses posterolaterally. In approximately 15% of the population, the external carotid artery originates lateral to the internal carotid artery. This anatomic variation occurs more frequently on the right (3:1). Carotid arteriography has shown that the proximal external carotid artery lies lateral to the internal carotid artery in 18% of the right bifurcations, and in 6% of the left.

There are eight named branches of the external carotid artery: the superior thyroid, ascending pharyngeal, lingual, facial, occipital, posterior auricular, and the terminal branches, the superficial temporal, and the maxillary artery.

The abundant number of anastomoses between the branches of the ECA and the intracranial circulation underscores its clinical significance as a collateral pathway for cerebral perfusion when significant disease is present in the internal carotid artery. Although there are many potential ECA-ICA anastomoses, blood flow from pterygopalatine branches of the maxillary artery to ethmoidal branches of the ophthalmic artery, and then to the supraclinoid ICA is the most frequent pattern. Other collateral pathways are from the branches of the superficial temporal artery to the internal carotid artery, the maxillary artery (middle meningeal) to lacrimal branches of the ophthalmic artery, and the facial artery branches through its orbital anastomoses.

Internal Carotid Artery[16-23]

The internal carotid artery is usually the larger terminal branch of the common carotid artery. The paired internal carotid arteries provide most of the blood supply to the frontal, temporal, and parietal lobes of the brain. The internal carotid artery is divided into four main segments: the cervical, petrous, cavernous, and the cerebral, or terminal ICA.

The cervical portion of the internal carotid artery begins at the common carotid bifurcation and extends to the base of the skull. The ICA lies in the carotid sheath and runs deep to the sternocleidomastoid muscle. In the majority of individuals, the internal carotid artery lies posterolateral to the external carotid artery and courses medially as it ascends in the neck. At its origin the cervical internal carotid artery normally has a slight dilation, termed the carotid bulb and/or the carotid sinus. The cervical ICA usually does not have branches. With age and progressive disease the internal carotid artery may become tortuous, coiled or kinked.

The internal carotid artery enters the skull through the carotid canal, which is just anterior to the jugular foramen in the petrous portion of the temporal bone. This is termed the petrous segment of the internal carotid artery. It runs vertically from the skull base for approximately one centimeter and then courses horizontally in an anteromedial direction. It emerges near the apex of the petrous temporal bone and curves above the cartilage occupying the foramen lacerum, where it ascends to a juxtasellar location piercing the dural layers of the cavernous sinus.

The internal carotid artery ascends within the cavernous sinus, and this third part is termed the cavernous segment. The artery courses slightly medially toward the posterior clinoid process. The ICA then runs anteriorly and horizontally lateral to the wall of the sphenoid sinus. This segment of the ICA terminates by ascending medial to the anterior clinoid process where it perforates the dura mater to enter the subarachnoid space. The "*S*" curvature of the internal carotid artery is referred to as the carotid siphon. The siphon is divided into three segments; the parasellar, the genu, and the supraclinoid.

The cerebral (supraclinoid) segment begins as the internal carotid artery emerges from the dura mater just below the optic nerve. The artery then courses superiorly and slightly laterally towards the lateral aspect of the optic chiasm and continues anteriorly. Just below the anterior perforated substance (medial end of the Sylvian fissure) it bifurcates into its two terminal branches, the anterior cerebral artery and the middle cerebral artery, which is usually the larger terminal branch. This segment of the ICA gives origin to the ophthalmic artery, the posterior communicating artery, and the anterior choroidal artery.

Ophthalmic Artery

The ophthalmic artery (OA) is the first branch of the internal carotid artery in the cerebral segment. It courses anterolateral and slightly downward through the optic foramen to supply the globe, orbit, and adjacent structures. The ophthalmic artery has three major groups of branches: the ocular branches, the orbital branches, and the extraorbital branches. The supraorbital artery, one of the ophthalmic artery's extraorbital branches travels from its origin and exits through the supraorbital foramen where it anastomoses with the superficial temporal artery. Theophthalmic artery terminates by dividing into a superior branch, the supratrochlear, and an inferior branch, the dorsal nasal, which anastomose with the superficial temporal and the facial arteries respectively. The branches of the ophthalmic artery often play an important role in collateral pathways that form as a result of disease of either the internal or external carotid arteries.

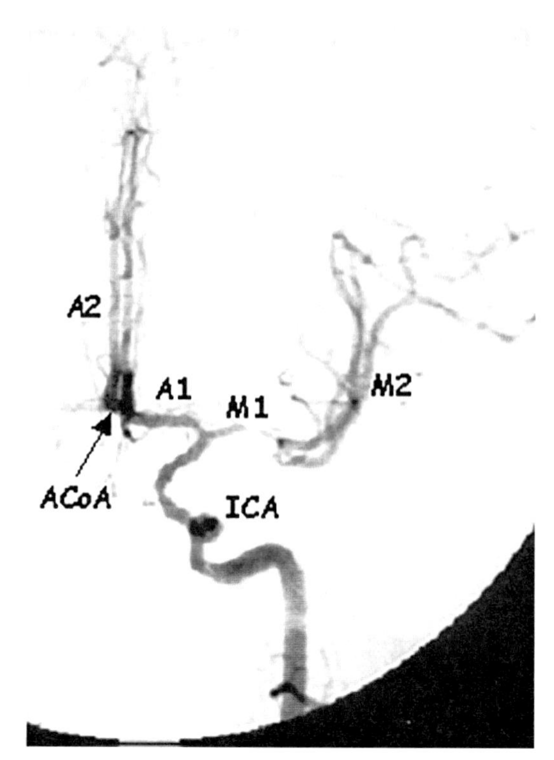

Figure 2-3. The anterior circulation of the circle of Willis. Anterior communicating artery (ACoA); Internal carotid artery (ICA); segments of the middle cerebral artery (M1 and M2); segments of the anterior cerebral artery (A1 and A2).

Posterior Communicating Artery[24-26]

The posterior communicating artery (PCoA) courses posteriorly and medially from theinternal carotid artery to join the posterior cerebral artery (PCA). The posterior communicating artery is variable in size and may angle upward or downward. It can be large when the P1 segment of the posterior cerebral artery is hypoplastic, which occurs in 15-22% of the cases. When the PCA is supplied from the ICA, this anatomic variant is termed a "*fetal*" origin of the posterior cerebral artery. Infrequently, the fetal origin circulation may also supply the last third of the basilar artery via the persistent trigeninal artery.

The posterior communicating artery is usually a potential rather than an actual arterial conduit. The PCoA generally does not function as an important collateral pathway unless the patient has extensive extracranial occlusive disease bilaterally or incomplete anterior cross-filling via the anterior communicating artery.

Middle Cerebral Artery[27-38]

The larger (diameter and length) terminal branch of the internal carotid artery is the middle cerebral artery (MCA), which is the blood supply to most of the lateral surface of the cerebral hemisphere (Figure 2-3). From its origin, the MCA extends laterally and horizontally in the lateral cerebral fissure. The horizontal segment may course downward or upward. The MCA either bifurcates or trifurcates prior to the limen insulae (a small gyrus) where the branches turn upward into the Sylvian fissure forming its genu ("knee"). The vessels course around the island of Reil, which is a triangular-shaped mound of cortex, and run postero-superiorly within the Sylvian fissure. The terminal branches of the MCA anastomose with terminal branches of the anterior cerebral and the posterior cerebral arteries.

The middle cerebral artery is usually divided into three segments. The main horizontal section from its origin to limen insulae is the M1 segment. This segment of the MCA gives rise to numerous, small lenticulostriate, or perforating branches. These vessels supply subcortical structures. The M2 segment is composed of the larger branches overlying the insular surface, and the segment exiting to the external cortical surface is called M3.

The initial MCA bifurcation is the third most common site for congenital aneurysms, giving rise to approximately one-fourth of all intracranial aneurysms. The anterior communicating and posterior communicating arteries are the first and second most common sites for aneurysm formation respectively. The MCA can also be the site for arterial stenosis and occlusion.

Anterior Cerebral Artery[39-52]

The anterior cerebral artery (ACA), is the smaller of the two terminal branches of the internal carotid artery. From its origin, the ACA courses antero-medially over the optic chiasm and optic nerve to the interhemispheric fissure (longitudinal cerebral fissure). The proximal, horizontal segment of the anterior cerebral artery is known as the A1 segment and is connected to the contralateral A1 segment via the anterior communicating artery. These vessels complete the anterior portion of the circle of Willis, and are part of a complete TCD evaluation.

The contour of the A1 segment may take a horizontal course, ascend or slightly descend. Complete absence of the A1 segment is unusual. An anomalous origin of the anterior cerebral artery is rare, but asymmetry between the two A1 segments is common. An inverse correlation exists between sizes of the A1 segment and the size of the anterior communicating artery. A small or hypoplastic A1 is usually found in conjunction with a large ACoA since the contralateral A1 segment supplies most of the blood flow to both distal ACA territories. Individuals with anomalies of the A1 segment have a slightly higher incidence of anterior communicating artery aneurysms. The anterior cerebral artery is a rare site for an isolated stenosis or occlusion.

Distal to the anterior communicating artery, the anterior cerebral arteries turn superiorly and run side by side in the interhemispheric fissure. The ACA curves around the genu of the corpus callosum in a postero-superior arc and runs posteriorly along its upper surface. The segment of the ACA from the anterior communicating artery to the distal anterior cerebral artery bifurcation (callosomarginal artery and pericallosal artery) is termed the A2 segment. The distal A2 segments anastomose with branches of the posterior cerebral arteries. A large medial striate artery, the recurrent artery of Heubner, is a major branch of the proximal A2 segment in approximately 80% of the cases, but this artery can also originate from the distal A1 segment.

Anterior Communicating Artery

The anterior communicating artery (ACoA) is a short vessel that connects the anterior cerebral arteries (A1) at the interhemispheric fissure. The ACoA may be absent, be a single, duplicated, or multi-channeled system. The longer anterior communicating arteries frequently are found to be curved, tortuous or kinked. The ACoA often is the location for congenital anomalies. The ACoA frequently is a site for aneurysm formation, and is the most common site of aneurysms associated with subarachnoid hemorrhage.

POSTERIOR CIRCULATION

Vertebral Artery[53-56]

The vertebral arteries (VA) are large branches of the subclavian arteries. Atherosclerotic changes usually occur at the origin of the vertebral arteries. The two vertebral arteries are equal in size in approximately 10% of the cases therefore size asymmetry is common. In the majority of cases, the left vertebral artery is the dominant artery. The vertebral artery can be divided into four segments: the extravertebral, intervertebral, horizontal, and the intracranial.

The extravertebral segment (VA1) courses superiorly and medially from its subclavicular origin to enter the transverse foramen of the sixth cervical vertebra. The proximal segment of the vertebral artery is approximately 4-5 cm in length and usually there are no branches. Anatomic variation of this segment occurs in about 10% and involve its entry in the third, fourth, fifth, or seventh cervical vertebra.

The intervertebral segment (VA2) ascends within the transverse foramina of the upper cervical vertebrae. As it reaches the C2 level it angles supero-laterally to the foramen of the axis, which is the second cervical vertebra. The vertebral artery then courses upward to the transverse foramen of the atlas, the first cervical vertebra. Branches from the intervertebral segment of the vertebral artery supply blood to the spinal arteries, and other branches anastomose with branches of the external carotid and subclavian arteries.

The horizontal segment (VA3) of the vertebral artery begins as it emerges from the transverse foramen of the atlas. The vessel curves posteriorly and medially around the articular process of the atlas and lies in a horizontal groove on the upper surface of the posterior arch of the atlas. It then angles anteriorly to enter the intraspinal canal, where small meningeal branches arise.

The intracranial portion (VA4) of the vertebral artery begins as it pierces the spinal dura and arachnoid immediately below the base of the skull at the foramen magnum (Figure 2-4). It continues medially and unites with the contralateral vertebral artery to form the basilar artery. Several major branches arise from this segment of the vertebral artery, the posterior and anterior spinal arteries, and the posterior inferior cerebellar artery (PICA), which is the largest branch of

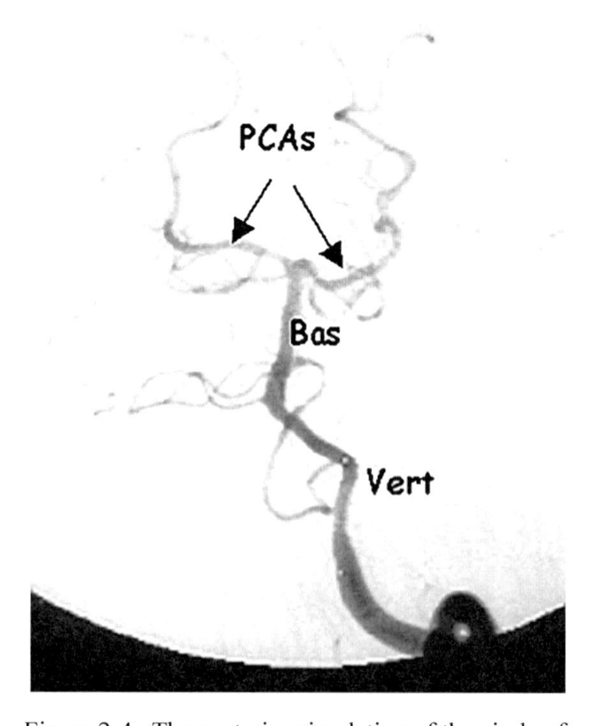

Figure 2-4. The posterior circulation of the circle of Willis. Vertebral artery (Vert); Basilar artery (Bas); Posterior cerebral artery (PCAs).

the vertebral artery. The PICA commonly arises approximately 1 - 2 cm proximal to the junction of the two vertebral arteries, however its origin varies, and is absent in approximately 15-20% of the population.

Basilar Artery[57]

The basilar artery (BA) is formed by the union of the two vertebral arteries, and is variable in its course, size, and length (2 – 3.5 cm). It usually originates at the lower border of the pons, extends anteriorly and superiorly and terminates by dividing into the paired posterior cerebral arteries. During its course the basilar artery gives off several branches including; the anterior inferior cerebellar artery (AICA), the internal auditory (labyrinthine) artery, the pontine branches, and the superior cerebellar arteries (SCA) just proximal to the posterior cerebral arteries. The basilar artery is often tortuous. Rarely, it may be duplicated or fenestrated.

Posterior Cerebral Artery[58-6]

The posterior cerebral arteries (PCA) originate from the terminal basilar artery and course anteriorly and laterally. The segment of PCA from its origin to its junction with the posterior communicating artery is termed P1, the pre-communicating portion. Many perforating branches that supply the brainstem and thalamus originate from this segment.

The portion of the vessel extending posteriorly from the PCoA to the posterior aspect of the midbrain is the P2 (ambient) segment, while the P3 segment continues posteriorly to the calcarine fissure. The PCA however, often divides into its terminal branches before reaching the calcarine fissure, and the P3 segment can be very short or nonexistent.

The proximal portion of the PCA is usually asymmetrical. In cases of a "fetal" origin, the P1 segment is hypoplastic or smaller than the PCoA. It is uncommon for occlusive disease to be limited to the PCA, but if it does occur, the P2 segment is most commonly affected.

Circle of Willis[63-74]

Sir Thomas Willis first described the circle of Willis in 1664. The circle is composed of the A1 segments of the two ACAs, the ACoA, the two PCoAs, the two ICAs, and the P1 segment of the two PCAs. It is a polygonal-shaped anastomotic ring at the base of the brain that permits shunting of blood between the right and left cerebral hemispheres (by the ACoA), and between the anterior and posterior systems (by the PCoAs). These communications are important when there is significant disease or occlusion of one of the major cervical arteries.

Variations of the circle of Willis are common. A classic "normal" circle of Willis is found in only approximately 20% of the cases. Significant hypoplasia or absence of the PCoA, ACoA, ACA (A1), and PCA (P1) are the most common variations.

Vessel Size

Observations indicate that the average diameter of the common carotid artery is 6-7 mm, the extracranial internal carotid artery is 5-6 mm, and the external carotid artery is 3-4 mm.

Intracranial arterial size information is summarized in Table 2-1. This information is compiled from several cadaver and angiographic analyses. Although cadaver and angiographic studies have their limitations, the approximation of vessel diameters is useful for understanding the intracranial anatomy and its relationship to the TCD examination. Additionally, the circle of Willis occupies the space that is approximately the size of a half dollar coin.

Table 2-1. Intracranial arterial diameters

Artery	Diameter (mm)	
	Average	Range
MCA (M1)	3.9	2.4 - 4.6
ACA (A1)	2.6	0.9-4.0
ACoA	1.5	0.2-3.4
Recurrent Artery of Heubner	0.8	0.3-1.5
PCA (P1)	2.6	0.8 –3.8
PCA (fetal)	1.8	0.8 -2.8
ICA (above PCoA)	4.3	2.5 -7.0
Ophthalmic	1.4	0.4 -2.0
Vertebral	2.2	1.5 -3.6
Basilar	4.1	3.0 -5.5

Intracranial Veins[75-81]

The veins of the cranium are divided into four groups: the cerebral, the sinuses of the dura mater, the diploic veins, and the emissary veins.

The veins draining the brain are tributaries of the venous sinuses that subsequently flow into the internal jugular veins. These veins are extremely thin walled, contain no valves, and are divided into three subcategories. The veins of the brain are: the cerebral veins (external and internal), the cerebellar veins (superior and inferior), and the veins of the brainstem.

The sinuses of the dura mater are venous channels that drain blood from the brain and the bones of the cranial cavity into the internal jugular vein. These veins are situated between the two layers of the dura mater and contain no valves. The sinuses of the dura mater are subdivided into two major groups; the posterosuperior sinuses and the anteroinferior sinuses.

The diploic veins (frontal, anterior temporal, posterior temporal, occipital) drain the diplöe of the cranial bones. These veins are irregular and have pouch-like dilatations. The emissary veins establish anastomoses between the skull and the veins on the exterior of the skull.

Doppler signals from the intracranial veins can be detected during a TCD examination. Intracranial venous Doppler signals are usually pulsatile, but they are less pulsatile than intracranial arterial signals. Although a detailed anatomic description of the intracranial veins is beyond the scope of this book, it is important for the TCD operator to know that Doppler signals from the intracranial veins may be detected during a TCD examination.

Summary

The description of anatomy in this chapter focused on the basal cerebral arteries evaluated during a TCD examination. To perform accurate TCD examinations, it is critical that the operator be familiar with the location of these arteries and the potential collateral pathways that may be evoked in the presence of disease.

References

Skull and Brain

1. Gray H. Gray's Anatomy 30th ed. Clemente CD (ed), Philadelphia: Lea & Febiger; Chapter 4, The Skull 1973: 158-225.

2. Gray H. Gray's Anatomy 30th ed. Clemente CD (ed), Philadelphia: Lea & Febiger; Chapter 11, Gross anatomy of the central nervous system, 1973: 957-1148.

3. Hollinshead WH. Textbook of Anatomy. 3rd ed. Philadelphia:Harper & Row; Chapter 25, skull, face and jaws, and Chapter 26,The cranial parts of the nervous system, 1974: 788-880.

4. Grolimund P: Transmission of ultrasound through the temporal bone. Chapter 2. In: Aaslid R (ed), Transcranial Doppler Sonography, New York: Springer-Verlag, 1986: 10-21.

5. White DN, Curry GR, Stevenson RJ. The acoustic characteristics of the skull. Ultrasound Med Biol 1978;4:225-252.

6. Eden A. Effect of emitted power on waveform intensity in transcranial Doppler. Stroke 1994;24:523-524.

7. Stolz E, Kaps M, Kern A, Dorndorf W. Frontal bone windows for transcranial color-coded duplex sonography. Stroke 1999;30(4):814-20.

Aortic Arch

8. Gray H. Gray's Anatomy 30th ed. Clemente CD (ed), Philadelphia: Lea & Febiger; Chapter 8, The arteries; The Aorta. 1973:662-665.

9. Bosniak MA. An analysis of some anatomic-roentgenologic aspects of the brachiocephalic vessels. AJR 1964;91: 1222-1231.

10. Lippert H, Pabst R. Arterial Variations in Man. Classification and Frequency, New York: Springer-Verlag, 1985:4-9.

11. Pakula H, Szapiro J. Anatomical studies of the collateral blood supply to the brain and upper extremity. J Neurosurg 1970;32:171-179.

12. Osborn AG. Introduction to cerebral angiography. Philadelphia: Harper & Row; Chapter 2, The aortic arch and its branches, 1980:33-48.

Common Carotid Artery

13. Gray H. Gray's Anatomy 30th ed. Clemente CD (ed), Philadelphia: Lea & Febiger; Chapter 8, The arteries; The common carotid artery, 1973:666-668.

External Carotid Artery

14. Teal JS, Rumbaugh CL, Bergeron RT, Segall HD. Lateral position of the external carotid artery: a rare anomaly? Radiology 1973;108:77-81.

15. Osborn AG. Introduction to cerebral angiography. Philadelphia: Harper & Row; Chapter 3, The external carotid artery, 1980:49-86.

Internal Carotid Artery

16. Gray H. Gray's Anatomy 30th ed. Clemente CD (ed), Philadelphia: Lea & Febiger; Chapter 8, The arteries; The internal carotid artery, 1973:682-688.

17. Gabrielsen TO, Greitz T. Normal size of the internal carotid, middle cerebral and anterior cerebral arteries. Acta Radiol 1970;10:1-10.

18. Gibo H, Lenkey C, Rhoton AL. Microsurgical anatomy of the supraclinoid portion of the internal carotid artery. J Neurosurg 1981;55:560-574.

19. Milenkovic Z. Anastomosis between internal carotid artery and anterior cerebral artery with other anomalies of the circle of Willis in a fetal brain. J Neurosurg 1981;55:701-703.

20. Paullus WS, Pait TG, Rhoton AL. Microsurgical exposure of the petrous portion of the carotid artery. J Neurosurg 1977;47:713-726.

21. Wollschlaeger PB, Wollschlaeger G. Anterior cerebral/internal carotid artery and middle cerebral/internal carotid artery ratios. Acta Radiol 1966;5:615-620.

22. Osborn AG. Introduction to cerebral angiography. Philadelphia: Harper & Row, Chapter 4, The internal carotid artery: cervical and petrous portions,1980:87-108

23. Osborn AG. Introduction to cerebral angiography. Philadelphia: Harper & Row; Chapter 5, The internal carotid artery: cavernous and supraclinoid portions, 1980:109-142.

Posterior Communicating Artery

24. Gray H. Gray's Anatomy 30th ed. Clemente CD (ed), Philadelphia: Lea & Febiger; Chapter 8, The arteries;The posterior communicating artery, 1973:692.

25. Bisaria KK. Anomalies of the posterior communicating artery and their potential clinical significance. J Neurosurg 1984; 60: 572-576.

26. Pedroza A, Dujovny M, Artero JC, et al. Microanatomy of the posterior communicating artery. Neurosurgery 1987;20: 228-235.

Middle Cerebral Artery

27. Gray H. Gray's Anatomy 30th ed. Clemente CD (ed), Philadelphia: Lea & Febiger; Chapter 8, The arteries; The middle cerebral artery, 1973:691-693

28. DeLong WB. Anatomy of the middle cerebral artery: The temporal branches. Stroke 1973;4:412-418.

29. Gabrielsen TO, Greitz T. Normal size of the internal carotid, middle cerebral and anterior cerebral arteries. Acta Radiol 1970;10:1-10.

30. Gibo H, Carver CC, Rhoton AL, et al. Microsurgical anatomy of the middle cerebral artery. J Neurosurg 1981; 54:151-169.

31. Marinkovic SV, Kovacevic MS, Marinkovic JM. Perforating branches of the middle cerebral artery: Microsurgical anatomy of their extracerebral segments. J Neurosurg 1985;63:266-271.

32. Ring BA. Middle cerebral artery: Anatomical and radiographic study. Acta Radiol 1962;57:289-300.

33. Teal JS, Rumbaugh CL, Bergeron RT, Segall HD. Anomalies of the middle cerebral artery: accessory artery, duplication, and early bifurcation. AJR 1973;118:567-575.

34. Umansky F, Juarez SM, Dujovny M, et al. Microsurgical anatomy of the proximal segments of the middle cerebral artery. J Neurosurg 1984; 61:458-467.

35. Umansky F, Dujovny M, Ausman JI, et al. Anomalies and variations of the middle cerebral artery: a microanatomical study. Neurosurgery 1988;22:1023-1027.

36. Umansky F, Gomes FB, Dujovny M, et al. The perforating branches of the middle cerebral artery. A microanatomical study. J Neurosurg 1985;62:261-268.

37. Watanabe T, Togo M. Accessory middle cerebral artery: Report of four cases. J Neurosurg 1974;41:248-251.

38. Osborn AG. Introduction to cerebral angiography. Philadelphia: Harper & Row; Chapter 9, The middle cerebral artery, 1980:239-294.

Anterior Cerebral and Anterior Communicating Arteries

39. Gray H. Gray's Anatomy 30th ed. Clemente CD (ed), Philadelphia: Lea & Febiger; Chapter 8, The arteries; The anterior cerebral artery, 1973:688-691.

40. Ahmed DS, Ahmed RH. The recurrent branch of the anterior cerebral artery. Anat Rec 1967;157:699-700.

41. Crowell RM, Morawetz RB. The anterior communicating artery has significant branches. Stroke 1977; 8:272-273.

42. Dunker RO, Harris AB. Surgical anatomy of the proximal anterior cerebral artery. Neurosurg 1976; 44:359-367.

43. Gacs G, Fox AJ, Barnett HJM, Vinuela F. Occurrence and mechanisms of occlusion of the anterior cerebral artery. Stroke 1983;14:952-959.

44. Gomes F, Dujovny M, Umansky F, et al. Microsurgical anatomy of the Recurrent Artery Of Heubner. J Neurosurg 1984;60:130-139.

45. Gomes FB, Dujovny M, Umansky F, et al. Microanatomy of the anterior cerebral artery. Surg Neurol 1986; 26:129-141.

46. Morris AA, Peck CM. Roentgenographic study of the variations in the normal anterior cerebral artery: One hundred cases studied in the lateral plane. AJR 1955;74:818-826.

47. Ostrowski AZ, Webster JE, Gurdjian ES. The proximal anterior cerebral artery: An anatomic study. Arch Neurol 1960;3:661-664.

48. Perlmutter D, Rhoton AL. Microsurgical anatomy of the anterior cerebral- anterior communicating- recurrent artery complex. J Neurosurg 1976;45:259-272.

49. Perlmutter D, Rhoton AL. Microsurgical anatomy of the distal anterior cerebral artery. J Neurosurg 1978;49:204-228.

50. Taren JA. Anatomical pathways related to the clinical findings in aneurysms of the anterior communicating artery. J Neurol Neurosurg Psychiat 1965;28:228-234.

51. Vincentelli F, Lehman G, Caruso G, et al. Extracerebral course of the perforating branches of the anterior communicating artery: microsurgical anatomical study. Surg Neurol 1991;35:98-104.

52. Osborn AG. Introduction to cerebral angiography. Philadelphia: Harper & Row; Chapter 7, The anterior cerebral artery, 1980:167-184.

Vertebral Artery and Basilar Artery

53. Gray H. Gray's Anatomy 30th ed. Clemente CD (ed), Philadelphia: Lea & Febiger; Chapter 8, The arteries; The vertebral artery and the basilar artery, 1973:696-702.

54. Lippert H, Pabst R. Arterial Variations in Man. Classification and Frequency, Springer-Verlag, New York, 1985:82.

55. Ross P, du Boulay G, Keller B. Normal measurements in angiography of the posterior fossa. Radiology 1975; 116:335-340.

56. Osborn AG. Introduction to cerebral angiography. Philadelphia: Harper & Row; Chapter 12, The arteries and the veins of the posterior fossa, 1980:379-427.

57. Haverling M. The tortuous basilar artery. Acta Radiol 1974;15:241-249.

Posterior Cerebral Artery

58. Gray H. Gray's Anatomy 30th ed. Clemente CD (ed), Philadelphia: Lea & Febiger; Chapter 8, The arteries; The posterior cerebral artery, 1973:701-703.

59. Ross P, du Boulay G, Keller B. Normal measurements in angiography of the posterior fossa. Radiology 1975; 116:335-340.

60. Saeki N, Rhoton AL. Microsurgical anatomy of the upper basilar artery and the posterior circle of Willis. J Neurosurg 1977;46: 563-578.

61. Williams DJ. The origin of the posterior cerebral artery. Brain 1936; 59:175-180.

62. Zeal AA, Rhoton AL. Microsurgical anatomy of the posterior cerebral artery. J Neurosurg 1978;48: 534-559.

Circle of Willis

63. Gray H. Gray's Anatomy 30th ed. Clemente CD (ed), Philadelphia: Lea & Febiger; Chapter 8, The arteries; The Circle of Willis, 1973:693-694.

64. Alpers BJ, Berry RG, Paddison RM. Anatomical studies of the circle of Willis in normal brain. Arch Neurol Psychiat 1959;81:409-418.

65. Alpers BJ, Berry RG. Circle of Willis in cerebral vascular disorders. The anatomical structure. Arch Neurol 1963;8:398-402.

66. Battacharji SK, Hutchinson EC, McCall AJ. The circle of Willis- The incidence of developmental abnormalities in normal and infarcted brains. Brain 1965;110:747-758.

67. Fisher CM. The Circle of Willis: Anatomical Variations. Vascular Diseases 1965;2:99-105.

68. Kayembe KNT, Sasahara M, Hazama F. Cerebral aneurysms and variations in the circle of Willis. Stroke 1984;15:846-850.

69. Lippert H, Pabst R. Arterial Variations in Man: Classification and Frequency, Springer-Verlag, New York, 1985:92-93.

70. Milenkovic Z. Anastomosis between internal carotid artery and anterior cerebral artery with other anomalies of the circle of Willis in a fetal brain. J Neurosurg 1981;55:701-703.

71. Pallie W, Samarasinghe DD. A study in the quantification of the circle of Willis. Brain 1962;85:569-578.

72. Puchades-Orts A, Nombela-Gomez M, Ortuno-Pacheco G. Variation in form of circle of Willis: Some anatomical and embryological considerations. Anat Rec 1975;185:119-124

73. Riggs HE, Rupp C. Variation in form of circle of Willis. Arch Neurol 1963, 8:24-30.

74. Osborn AG. Introduction to cerebral angiography. Philadelphia: Harper & Row. Chapter 6, The Circle of Willis, 1980:143-166.

Veins

75. Gray H. Gray's Anatomy 30th ed. Clemente CD (ed), Philadelphia: Lea & Febiger; Chapter 9, The veins;Veins of the head and neck, 1973:799-820.

76. Bub B, Ferris EJ, Levy PS, Navani S. The Cerebral Venogram: a statistical analysis of the sequence of venous filling in cerebral angiograms. Radiology 1968;91:1112-1118.

77. Huang YP, Wolf BS. Veins of the white matter of the cerebral hemispheres (the medullary veins): Diagnostic importance in carotid angiography. AJR 92:739-755, 1964.

78. Huang YP, Wolf BS. The veins of the posterior fossa-superior or Galenic draining group. AJR 1965;95:808-821.

79. Newton TH, Potts DG (Ed) Radiology Of The Skull And Brain: Angiography. Veins, Volume 2, Book 3, C.V. Mosby Co., St. Louis, 1974.

80. Wolf BS, Huang YP. The insula and deep middle cerebral venous drainage system: Normal anatomy and angiography. AJR 1963;90:472-489.

81. Osborn AG. Introduction to cerebral angiography. Philadelphia: Harper & Row; Chapter 11, The veins of the head and neck, 1980:327-378.

General

Gray H. Gray's Anatomy 30th ed. Clemente CD (ed), Philadelphia: Lea & Febiger. Chapter 8, The arteries and Chapter 9, The veins 1973.

Kido DK, Baker RA, Rumbaugh CL: Normal Cerebral Vascular Anatomy. In: Abrams HL (Ed) Abrams Angiography. Vascular and Interventional Radiology. Third Edition. Boston: Little, Brown and Company, pp 231-270, 1983.

Lippert H, Pabst R. Arterial Variations In Man: Classification And Frequency. New York: Springer-Verlag, 1985.

Newton TH, Potts G (Ed). Radiology Of The Skull And Brain: Angiography. Arteries, Volume 2, Book 2, St. Louis: C.V. Mosby Co., 1974.

Osborn AG. Introduction to Cerebral Angiography. Philadelphia: Harper & Row, 1980.

Osborn AG. Diagnostic Neuroradiology. Philadelphia: Harper & Row, 1994.

Osborn AG. Diagnostic Cerebral Angiography. 2nd ed. Philadelphia: Lippincott Williams & Wilkins, 1998.

Stephens RB, Stilwell DL. Arteries And Veins Of The Human Brain. Charles C. Thomas, Springfield, Illinois, 1969.

Chapter 3
Transcranial DopplerTechnique

Considerable progress has been made in the transcranial Doppler (TCD) examination since its first description in 1982.[1] The most reliable and reproducible results are obtained by proper instrument control settings, careful patient positioning, proper utilization of the examination sites, and accurate vessel identification. Common problems can be avoided if the operator is aware of them and slightly modifies the technique. Once vessel identification is accurate and studies become reproducible, the operator will have confidence in the TCD results.

This chapter describes: 1) the equipment settings, 2) proper patient and operator position, 3) TCD examination sites, 4) technical aspects of intracranial artery identification, and 5) hints to reduce technical errors when performing TCD examinations.

Equipment

The TCD examination is performed using a 2 MHz, focused, pulsed Doppler transducer with the received ultrasound signal displayed as uni- or bi-directional spectral waveforms. A low frequency transducer decreases attenuation of the ultrasound wave caused by bone. Furthermore, using a smaller size transducer and a 1 MHz frequency may prove valuable when examining patients with small/poor TCD windows.[2,3] Although specifications vary between manufacturers, the conventional signal display shows blood flow toward the transducer above the zero baseline and blood flow away from the transducer below the baseline. Spectral Doppler waveforms are displayed in real-time, and pertinent quantifications (i.e. mean velocity, pulsatility index) are calculated and automatically updated with each display sweep. These automated values are correct only if a flow signal with optimized signal-to-noise contrast is obtained. In addition, several post-processing quantifications can be obtained automatically or manually after freezing the spectral waveforms (i.e. peak systolic velocity, end diastolic velocity, pulsatility index, etc). A good quality transcranial Doppler examination depends upon the proper adjustment of several instrument controls (power, gain, etc.) and is defined by each individual patient's cerebral hemodynamics.

The real time display of all the Doppler shift frequencies over time is the Doppler spectral waveform. Time (seconds) is recorded along the horizontal axis, and velocity (frequency) is on the vertical axis. Velocity is recorded in centimeters per second (cm/sec). The velocity scale is divided by a zero baseline, with a positive Doppler shift (toward the transducer) displayed above the baseline, and a negative Doppler shift (away from the transducer) below the baseline. Accurate recording of the intracranial arterial Doppler spectral waveforms is critical, since this is the basis for the interpretation of the transcranial Doppler examination. At each sample volume depth, the operator usually should not settle for the first signal located, but instead should take the time to angle the transducer to obtain the best quality Doppler signal.

Sample volume size

The sample volume is the specific anatomic area from which the pulsed Doppler echoes are accepted by the equipment. In other words, blood flowing within the sample volume generates the Doppler shifts detected by the ultrasound equipment. During TCD examinations, the sample volume depth will vary as the different intracranial arteries are evaluated. The sample volume size used during a TCD examination is usually from 10-15 mm for the best sensitivity and signal-to-noise ratio.

Using a large Doppler sample volume size to evaluate the small intracranial arteries causes two effects on the spectral Doppler waveform. First, the sample volume size is larger than the diameter of any intracranial artery. Thus, the Doppler shift will contain the fast moving blood flow from the center of the vessel's lumen and the slow moving blood flow along the walls of the artery. Because the sample volume includes the blood flow from the entire lumen of the artery, all TCD Doppler spectral waveforms will demonstrate spectral broadening. Thus, spectral broadening is not used as an interpretation criterion for TCD examinations. Second, the large sample volume size usually contains Doppler frequency shifts from more than one artery or from one artery and its branches. This may be displayed in the Doppler spectral waveform as blood flowing in both directions (toward and away from the transducer) or a Doppler signal from one artery with a more intense signal from a second artery displayed within the first artery's signal (Figure 3-1).

Doppler gain

The Doppler gain serves as an amplifier for the incoming Doppler signals. During a TCD study, it is important to adjust the Doppler gain so that the peak trace envelope, which is instrument dependent, accurately follows the peak velocity outline of the spectral waveform. Occasionally, amplification of weak Doppler signals produces considerable background noise and the peak trace envelope is inaccurate. When this occurs, the operator has to calculate the mean velocity by manually measuring the peak systolic and end diastolic velocities, or by visually estimating the mean velocity.

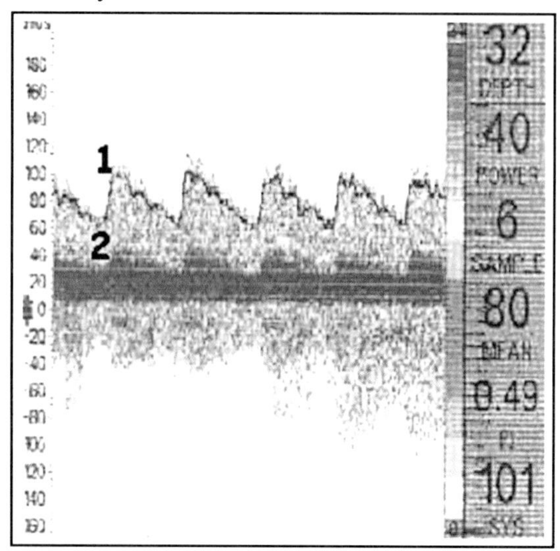

Figure 3-1. Doppler shift from two middle cerebral artery branches (1 and 2) displayed in one spectral waveform.

Pulse Repetition Frequency

The number of ultrasound pulses emitted by the transducer per second is the pulse repetition frequency (PRF). Higher Doppler shifts may be detected with a higher PRF (velocity scale). The upper limit to Doppler shifts that can be detected is one half of the PRF, the Nyquist limit. When the Nyquist limit is exceeded, aliasing occurs in the Doppler spectral waveform display, making it difficult to accurately calculate the mean velocity. To display increased velocities (eliminate aliasing), the operator can increase the velocity scale and/or decrease the zero baseline to increase the scale in one direction.

Doppler output/intensity

Safety issues concerning ultrasound that include thermal and the cavitational bioeffect mechanisms are related to Doppler output (intensity). The operator adjusts this control, and the various manufacturers display the values that measure output differently. The Doppler power should be increased to the maximum power setting for adequate penetration of the adult skull. However, it should be at the lowest level necessary and applied for the shortest duration as possible to obtain good clinical information. The ALARA ("as low as reasonably achievable") principle should be applied during TCD examinations. Acoustical intensity settings should be decreased to a minimum (10% or 17 mW/cm^2) when using the transorbital window.

M-mode

One transmitter (transducer) is used to generate a pulse and receive echoes arriving at different time intervals, or gates. Modern TCD units are equipped with either multi-gate displays or with power motion (M-mode) Doppler.[4] The latter provides real-time spatial display of blood flow direction and intensity from 33 overlapping gates, or sample volumes that cover 6.5 cm path of beam propagation (Figure 3-2 A, B). M-mode is a display presenting a spot brightening for each echo voltage delivered from the receiver. This produces a two-dimensional recording of the reflector position (depth) versus time. Time is displayed along the horizontal axis and depth along the vertical axis. This format may also be color coded for the direction of blood flow. The display is red for blood flow toward the transducer and is color-coded blue for blood flow away from the transducer.

The use of M-mode in the TCD examination permits the visualization of hemodynamic information from multiple depths at the same time. This may potentially be useful in locating the ultrasound window, allowing rapid assessment of directionality changes during monitoring, and may increase the accuracy of detecting emboli.[5] M-mode helps the operator to select a depth for single gate spectral interrogation similar to color flow imaging of the extracranial carotid system.

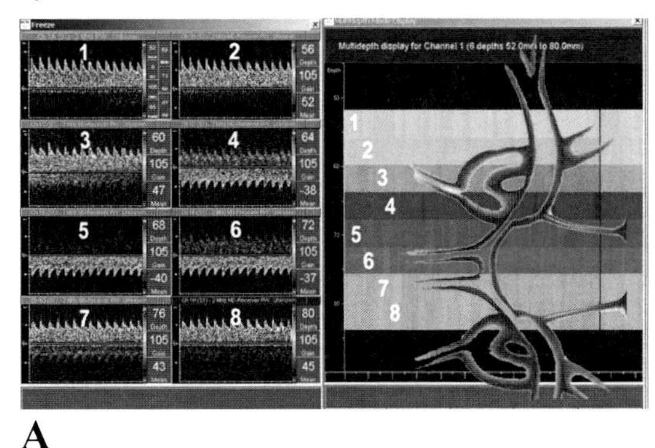

A

B

Figure 3-2 A, B. Two examples of M-Mode color TCD. [Courtesy of Nicolet Vascular and Spencer Technologies]

Doppler spectral waveforms

The Doppler spectral waveforms recorded during a TCD examination are similar to those obtained from the cervical internal carotid artery (ICA). Diastolic flow is present throughout the cardiac cycle because of the low peripheral resistance of the brain. Describing the spectral waveforms from the intracranial arteries, peak velocity refers to the highest velocity noted in systole, and end diastolic velocity is the maximal velocity just prior to the acceleration phase (systole) of the next waveform (Figure 3-3). During TCD examinations, however, mean velocity is the parameter reported. The preference to use mean velocity instead of peak systolic velocity for TCD examinations is because the mean velocity is less affected by systemic factors such as heart rate, contractility, total peripheral resistance, and it correlates better with perfusion.[6]

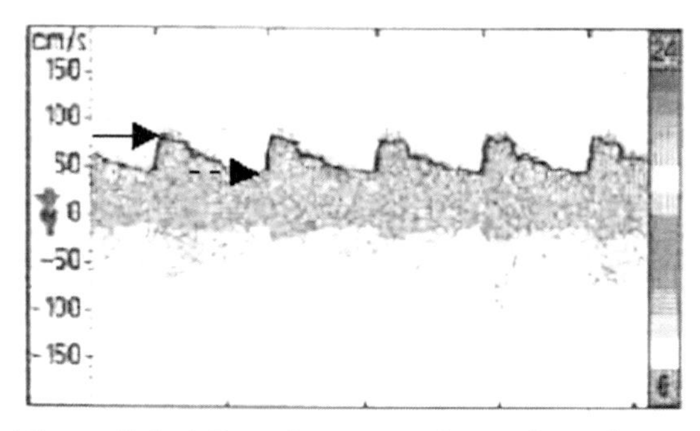

Figure 3-3. A Doppler spectral waveform from a middle cerebral artery. Peak systolic velocity is 82 cm/sec (solid arrow), end diastolic velocity is 44 cm/sec (dashed arrow), mean velocity is 59 cm/sec, and the pulsatility index is 0.65.

The mean velocity calculated by TCD equipment is based upon the time average of the outline velocity (maximum velocity envelope). The velocity envelope is a trace of the peak velocities as a function of time. The quality of the maximum velocity envelope is responsible for the accuracy of the instrument's calculation of the mean velocity and the pulsatility index (P.I.). The operator adjusts the Doppler gain and intensity levels to obtain the best signal-to-noise ratio. Improper gain adjustment or intensity settings result in unsatisfactory maximum velocity envelopes (Figure 3-4 A, B, C). If this occurs, the automatic calculations produced by the TCD equipment are invalid. The mean velocity can be estimated in these cases, however, by positioning the horizontal cursor at the velocity where the area below the peak velocity and above the cursor are equal to the area below the cursor and above the peak velocity envelope in diastole (Figure 3-5).

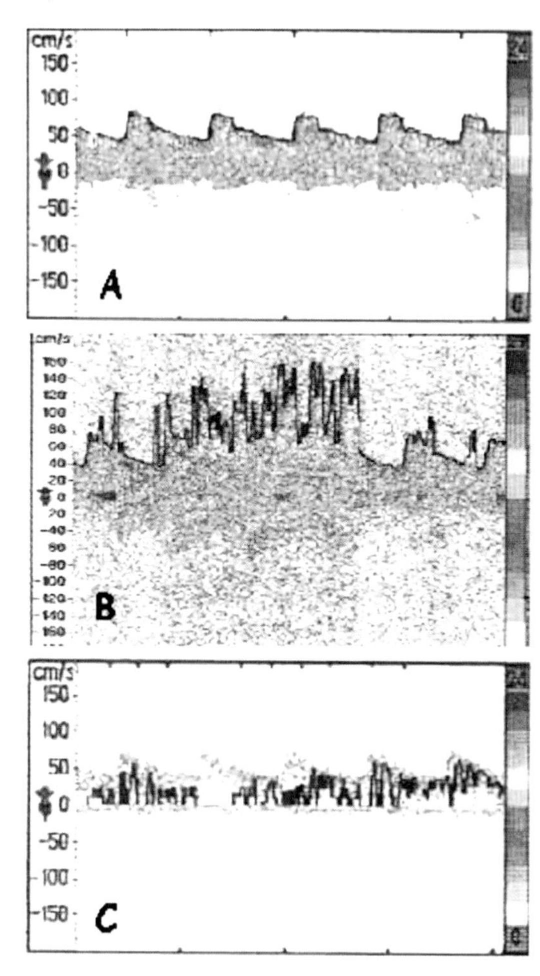

Figure 3-4. A Doppler spectral waveform from a middle cerebral artery with different gain settings.
A) Proper gain setting; mean velocity is 59 cm/sec and the pulsatility index is 0.65.
B) Increased gain setting; mean velocity is 76 cm/sec and the pulsatility index is 1.24.
C) Reduced gain setting; mean velocity is 19 cm/sec and the pulsatility index is 2.85.

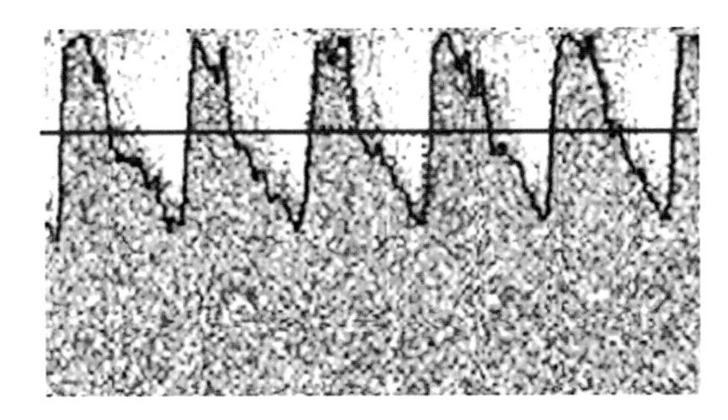

Figure 3-5. The horizontal cursor is placed so the area below the peak velocity and above the cursor is equal to the area below the cursor and above the peak velocity envelope in diastole.

Another method to estimate the mean velocity of a TCD Doppler signal is to use one of the following two formulas:

$$\frac{\text{(peak systolic - end diastolic)}}{3} + \text{end diastolic vel.}$$

or

$$\frac{\text{peak systolic + (end diastolic x2)}}{3}$$

Depending upon the manufacturing company, the maximum velocity envelope on TCD equipment may only be functional above the zero baseline. The values calculated with each display sweep apply only to the Doppler spectral waveforms that appear above the baseline. If blood flow is away from the transducer (below the baseline), it may be necessary to change the direction of the waveform on the display to above the baseline so that the equipment can perform the computations. It is important that the operator and interpreter be aware of the direction icon on the display that indicates whether blood flow is away from or toward the transducer.

Position

Patient

TCD examinations are performed with the patient in the supine position. An examination table is preferable, however, if the patient is immobile, s/he can be examined lying on a stretcher or in a hospital bed. The patient's neck should be straight with their head placed on a small pillow. Maintaining patient comfort cannot be overemphasized, since head movements are minimized which may change the transducer-artery angle. Respiratory changes due to anxiety are also reduced thereby avoiding hypercapnia or hypocapnia, which cause fluctuations in cerebral blood flow. Before beginning the examination, enough time should be allowed for the stabilization of the patient's heart rate and blood pressure.

The supine position allows access to the transtemporal, transorbital, and submandibular windows, whereas other positions are used for the suboccipital approach. The suboccipital examination can be performed with the patient lying supine and the head turned to one side, with the patient sitting and the head lowered slightly towards their chest, or with the patient lying on the side with the head bowed slightly so the chin touches their chest. We have found the suboccipital examination easier if the patient is able to tolerate lying on their side.

Operator

A good quality TCD examination requires concentration. Therefore, the operator should not be rushed or interrupted. Time, patience, and alert thinking are required for consistently accurate TCD examinations. The operator should be schooled in Doppler ultrasound principles, cerebrovascular hemodynamics, and intracranial anatomy, as well as appreciate the potential intracranial collateral blood flow patterns.

The operator sits near the patient's head and stabilizes the examining arm by resting the elbow on the examination table. This placement of the arm eliminates minor spontaneous hand movements that may cause intracranial arterial Doppler signals to be lost, and prevents motion artifact from being introduced into the signal. From this position, the operator also has equal access to both sides of the patient's head, permitting the best orientation of the transducer to the body.

It is critical that the operator maintains a comfortable and ergonomically sound position when performing TCD examinations.[7] Proper body mechanics and postural alignment will assist in avoiding pain and injury. It is important to have an easily adjustable examination table for the patient and an adjustable chair or stool for the operator. In addition, it is very important to support your arm when scanning, placing a pillow underneath your arm if necessary. Use a relaxed grip on the transducer. Remember that it is critical to your health to take a few minutes to find the proper position.

During bedside examinations, it is advantageous for the operator to position herself/himself behind the head of the bed. In some instances (i.e. intensive care units), it may be difficult for the operator to achieve this position. Whatever extra effort is exerted for proper positioning will be rewarded by improved results and will be helpful in minimizing unhealthy body positions. The optimal second choice is to stand on either side of the patient, resting the examining arm on the bed for stabilization. In this position the operator may find it more difficult to perceive the transducer-artery angle. During bedside examinations, the operator must always adjust her/his perception of the transducer-artery angle due to changes in her/his position. Additionally, bedside examinations will be technically easier to perform if the operator uses a remote control unit.

The use of stereo headphones is recommended when performing TCD examinations. Headphones eliminate extraneous noise, providing the operator the optimal environment to detect subtle changes associated with the Doppler signals during the TCD examination.

At the end of the examination, the ultrasound gel should be removed from the patient. Excess gel should be removed from the ultrasound transducer and it should be cleaned using a disinfectant.

Examination Sites

There are four ultrasound pathways ("windows") allowing access to the intracranial arteries. A complete standard TCD examination incorporates the following approaches:

1. **Transtemporal**
2. **Transorbital**
3. **Suboccipital**
4. **Submandibular**

The placement of the transducer for the four approaches is illustrated in Figure 3-6. The intracranial arteries evaluated by each approach are listed in Table 3-1. Technical hints used to locate the ultrasound windows are presented first, followed by a more detailed discussion of each TCD approach.

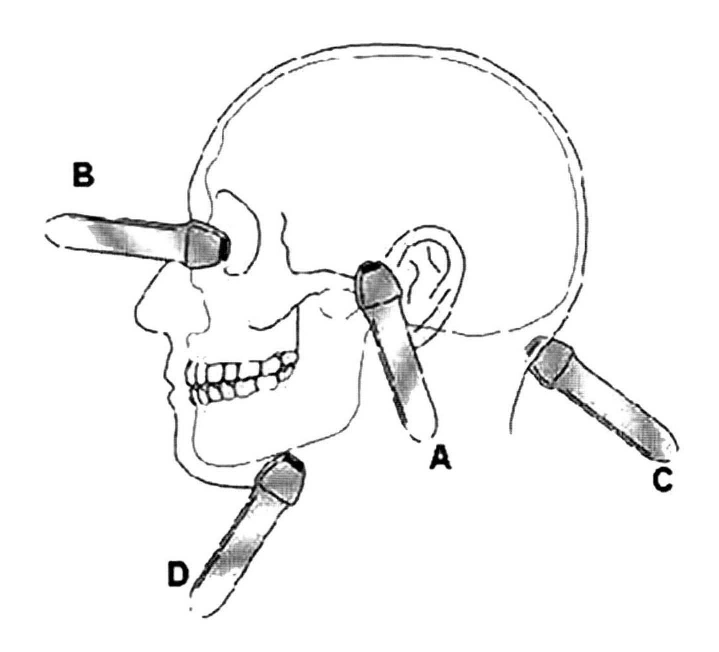

Figure 3-6. Transducer position is displayed for the four TCD windows. (A) transtemporal, (B) transorbital, (C) suboccipital, and (D) submandibular. [From: Katz ML. Intracranial Cerebrovascular Evaluation. In: Textbook of Diagnostic Ultrasonography. Mosby, St. Louis, 2001]

Table 3-1. The transcranial Doppler windows and the intracranial arteries.

Window	Artery
Transtemporal	Middle Cerebral
	Anterior Cerebral
	Anterior Communicating
	Terminal Internal Carotid
	Posterior Cerebral
	Posterior Communicating
Transorbital	Ophthalmic
	Internal Carotid (siphon)
Suboccipital	Vertebral
	Basilar
Submandibular	Internal Carotid

Ultrasound Windows

Finding the proper ultrasound window occasionally may be difficult and time consuming. The ultrasound beam needs to penetrate either the temporal bone or a natural cranial ostium, and to intercept the small intracranial arteries in a specific location. Time and patience are essential in identifying optimal TCD windows so that information will be received by the transducer and good quality Doppler spectral waveforms will be produced.

If a Doppler signal is located upon initial skin contact, then minimal movement or angling of the transducer maximizes the quality of the ultrasound signal. If a signal is not immediately appreciated, and the instrument control settings are correct, then several technical maneuvers can be performed.

Changing the angle of the transducer, thereby redirecting the ultrasound beam, often helps in locating an ultrasound window. The importance of angling the transducer becomes apparent when the variation in size, location, and tortuousity of the intracranial arteries are considered. When angling the transducer to obtain the best quality Doppler signal, part of the face of the transducer is often elevated off the surface of the skin. Additional ultrasound gel may be needed in these cases to maintain good transducer-gel contact.

Simply adjusting the location of the transducer is all that is needed in some patients to find a good ultrasound window. The transducer, however, should be moved slowly over the skin's surface. Moving the transducer 1-2 millimeters frequently finds the window and/or significantly improves the quality of the Doppler signal. Once window presence is noticed, an operator should stop moving the probe relative to skull surface and slowly adjust the transducer's angulation. While adjusting the transducer's position, good transducer-gel contact must be maintained.

The depth setting of the sample volume is another important parameter to adjust when trying to locate the ultrasound window. This will vary with each TCD approach. The depth setting should be adjusted to one that has a high probability of insonating the desired intracranial artery from the approach being used. Since there are differences in the size and shape of patients' heads, and variations of the intracranial arterial anatomy, the sample volume depth setting should be adjusted when searching for an optimal window. Most operators find that the combination of altering the transducer's angle and/or location, and the depth of the sample volume is very rewarding when trying to locate a TCD window.

As mentioned, good transducer-gel-skin contact is important, and can be maintained with minimal pressure by the transducer. Excessive pressure may create patient discomfort causing anxiety and movement, and may push the ultrasound gel from beneath the transducer causing the Doppler signal to be lost. Although extra pressure may be required to locate a small window in an elderly patient, once this window is located the pressure can be decreased to a minimum necessary to continue blood flow velocity tracking and at a level comfortable for the patient. Proper pressure eliminates interposed air and maintains gel contact between the transducer and skin. When performing TCD examinations, the patient's hair may also prevent good transducer-gel-skin contact. If a good Doppler signal is not obtained, additional ultrasound gel should be applied to compensate for this minor problem. At the end of the TCD examination, the ultrasound gel should be removed from the patient, and the ultrasound transducer should be cleaned with a disinfectant.

Transtemporal Window

The transtemporal approach provides the most information about the intracranial hemodynamics. Finding this window can be difficult, and at times frustrating, because ultrasound penetration of the temporal bone is required. Other windows used during a TCD examination are usually less difficult to locate because natural ostia allow easy intracranial penetration of the ultrasound beam.

The transtemporal window varies in size and location with each patient, and may vary in an individual from one side to the other. Attenuation of the Doppler signal occurs at the temporal bone interface and its magnitude depends on the thickness of the bone. Grolimund found that the power measured behind the skull was nevergreater than 35% of the transmitted power, and the mean value of the power loss was 80%.[8] The ability to penetrate the temporal bone is influenced by the patient's age, sex, and race.[8-12] Hyperostosis of the skull is commonly found in older individuals, females, and in African Americans. Even though the maximum acoustical intensity of the TCD equipment should be used when trying to locate the transtemporal window, it is still not found in approximately 10-30% of the population. Since the transducer is frequently in contact with the patient's hair during this approach, operators are reminded to use generous amounts of ultrasonic gel to maintain good transducer-gel contact when trying to locate the window.

The transtemporal approach has been described as being divided into three locations over the temporal bone: the anterior, mid, and posterior temporal windows (Figure 3-7).

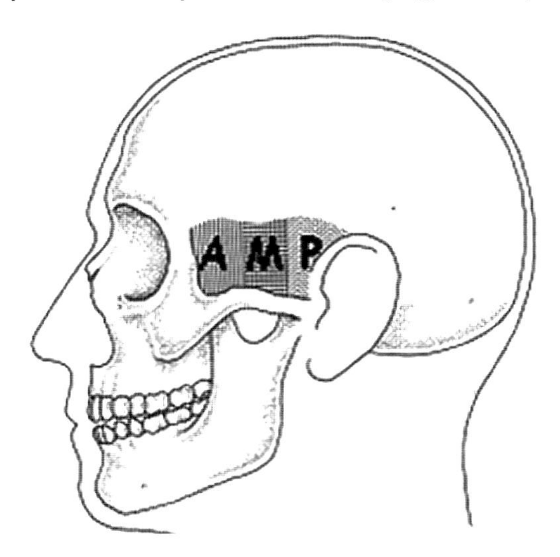

Figure 3-7. The anterior (A), mid (M), and posterior (P) locations for the transtemporal window. [From: Katz ML. Intracranial Cerebrovascular Evaluation. In: Textbook of Diagnostic Ultrasonography. Mosby, St. Louis, 2001]

The posterior transtemporal window is located superior to the zygomatic arch and anterior to the ear, with the transducer aimed in a slightly anterior direction. The anterior transtemporal window is just posterior to the frontal process of the zygoma, and a slight posterior angulation of the transducer is required for accurate insonation. The ultrasound beam is directed medially to properly access the mid transtemporal window, which is located between the anterior and posterior windows.

The mid and posterior transtemporal windows are used more frequently than the anterior window. The mid-transtemporal window is the ideal location because the terminal ICA bifurcation, which is the TCD reference signal, can be detected by aiming directly medial with the transducer. Each transtemporal window can be used to obtain accurate velocity data if the angle of the transducer is considered in searching for the intracranial arteries. It is important, therefore, to systematically evaluate the entire region so that good quality Doppler signals can be obtained from the best temporal position. It may also be useful during a TCD examination via the transtemporal window to change the position of the transducer to obtain the best Doppler signal from each of the intracranial arteries. If a transtemporal window is located on only one side of the patient, the contralateral arteries may be evaluated through this window. Evaluating the contralateral arteries from a transtemporal window may be difficult in many patients, and this technique should only be used when absolutely necessary.

A sample volume depth of 50-60 mm is used during the initial search for the transtemporal window because it offers the greatest likelihood of detecting the middle cerebral artery stem. The acoustical intensity level should be at 100% of its maximum during the search, and then set as low as possible without sacrificing the quality of the Doppler signal. The intensity level needed for the TCD examination varies between patients, may differ from side to side, and may need to be changed during the examination. The intensity level often needs to be increased as the deeper intracranial arteries are evaluated.

Once a Doppler signal is identified, the sampling depth should be adjusted to locate the terminal internal carotid artery (t-ICA) bifurcation. The origin of the middle cerebral artery (MCA) and the anterior cerebral artery (ACA) are located at the bifurcation of the t-ICA. The Doppler spectral waveform at this location is bi-directional (Figure 3-8). Blood flow in the MCA is toward the transducer and is displayed above the baseline, and blood flow in the ACA is away from the transducer and is displayed below the baseline. This signal is often referred to as the "butterfly" waveform. It should be noted that the Doppler signal from this location might be confusing to interpret because blood flow from the t-ICA (toward the transducer) may also be captured within the large sample volume. In fact, a TCD examination performed using a sample volume size of 10-15 mm covers the distance 3-5 times greater than a normal MCA diameter and appearance of bi-directional signals at varying depths should be expected. Reduction of sample volume size may help to focus on specific arterial segments.

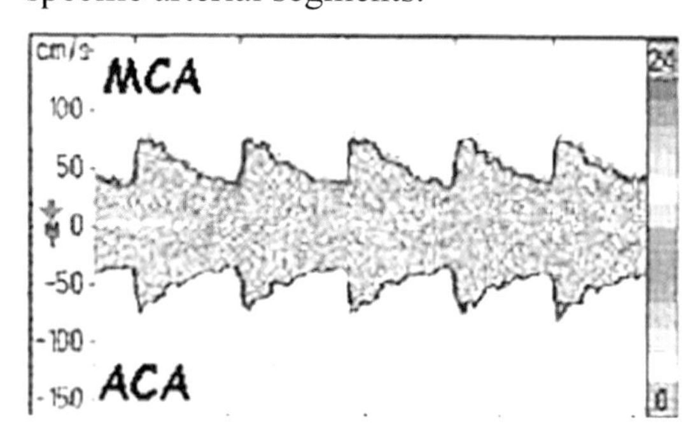

Figure 3-8. The terminal-internal carotid artery bifurcation Doppler signal obtained at a depth of 64 mm. Blood flow is above the baseline (toward the transducer) in the middle cerebral artery (MCA) and below the baseline (away from the transducer) in the anterior cerebral artery (ACA).

Although the depth of the t-ICA Doppler signal varies slightly with each patient, it is usually found in most adults between 60-67 mm. In a small percentage of patients, however, a t-ICA bifurcation signal may not be located due to an anatomic variation of the MCA and/or the ACA. In these cases, the reference point becomes the sample volume depth at which the MCA Doppler signal changes to the ACA signal.

When the t-ICA bifurcation has been located, adjusting the transducer's angle and position on the skin's surface optimizes the Doppler signal. Finding the best transtemporal window is important because this bi-directional signal is the critical landmark leading to accurate identification of the other intracranial arteries, and allows one to appreciate proper intracranial arterial spatial relationships.

Middle Cerebral Artery

Once the optimal t-ICA bifurcation signal is identified, the middle cerebral artery is examined by incremental reduction of the sample volume depth by 2-5 mm steps from the reference signal. At each depth setting, the angle of the transducer is adjusted to obtain the best quality Doppler signal. In this manner, it is possible to ultrasonically "trace" the anatomic route of the artery. In other words, the operator should "go with the flow", and re-adjust the transducer's position to properly display the Doppler signals with each consecutive change in the depth of insonation.

The MCA usually can be traced superficially to approximately 30-40 mm, and blood flow is normally toward the transducer (Figure 3-9 A, B, C). The MCA mean velocity is 62 $\pm$ 12 cm/sec.

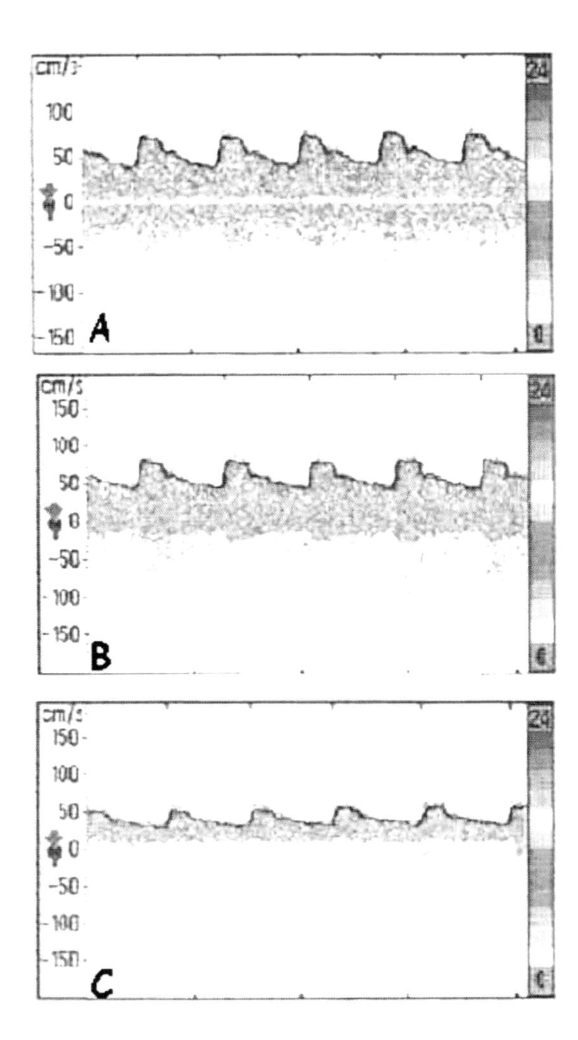

Figure 3-9. The middle cerebral artery signal is traced superficially from the terminal-ICA bifurcation. The MCA signal at, A) a depth of 60 mm; mean velocity is 54 cm/sec, B) a depth of 54 mm; mean velocity is 54 cm/sec, and C) a depth of 44 mm; mean velocity is 40 cm/sec.

Doppler signals can be obtained from the branches of the MCA at the superficial levels (30-45 mm), but often acquiring these signals requires severe modification of the transducer's angle. The distal MCA branches course superiorly and slightly posteriorly over the insula causing a greater angle of insonation that results in a lower velocity. The distal MCA branches (early anterior temporal or more distal M2 branches) may produce Doppler signals that are directed away from the transducer.

Anterior Cerebral Artery

After completing the MCA evaluation, the artery is retraced by increasing the sample volume depth, thereby returning to the t-ICA bifurcation. When the characteristic, bifurcation signal is relocated and optimized, the sample volume depth is increased by 2-5 mm in stepwise fashion to trace the ACA (A1 segment). The ACA usually can be identified if the transducer is aimed slightly anteriorly and superiorly from the t-ICA bifurcation. At each depth setting, it is important to adjust the angle of the transducer to obtain the best quality Doppler signal. Normally blood flow in the ACA is away from the transducer (Figure 3-10 A, B, C), and the mean velocity is 50 ± 11 cm/sec. The ACA is usually only followed for 1 to 3 sample volume depth steps because of its short length and anatomic pathway.

Since the ACA is smaller in diameter and often is tortuous, it is usually more difficult to detect and follow than the middle cerebral artery. The intensity level may need to be increased to obtain good quality Doppler signals from the ACA, which is located deeper than the MCA. Additionally, depending on the equipment being used, the direction of the signal may need to be inverted so that the waveform is displayed above the baseline for velocity measurements.

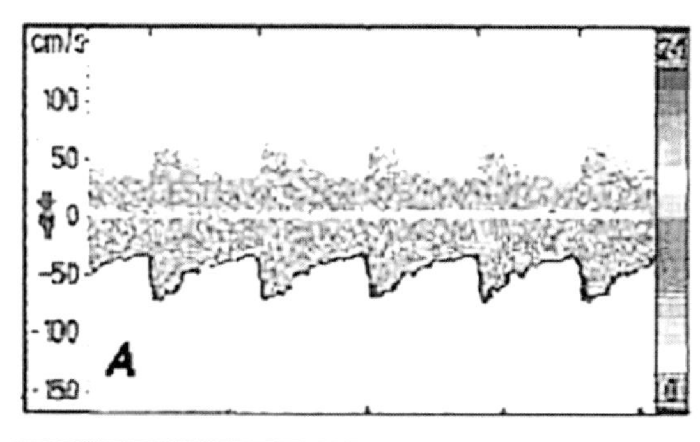

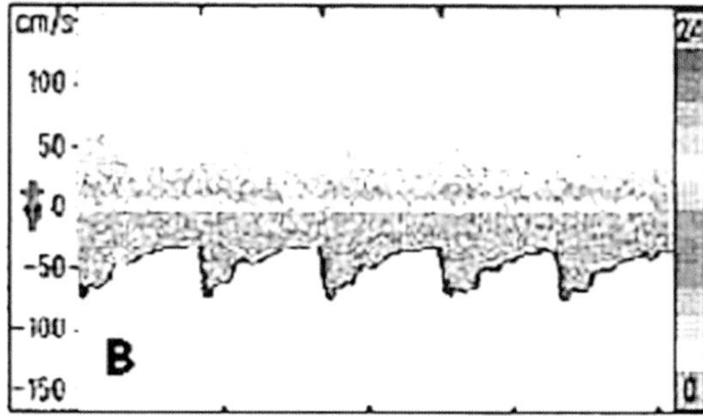

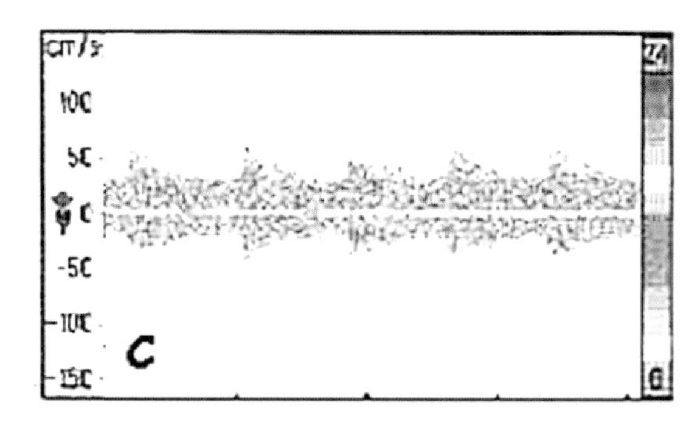

Figure 3-10. The anterior cerebral artery (ACA) Doppler signal is traced to the midline. The ACA at,A) a depth of 68 mm; mean velocity is 46 cm/sec, B) a depth of 72 mm; mean velocity is 44 cm/sec, and C) a depth of 80 mm the ipsilateral ACA is below the baseline and the contralateral ACA is above the zero baseline.

As the ACA is traced toward midline, another bi-directional signal is often encountered (Figure 3-10 C). Midline in most adults is between 70 and 80 mm. At this point, blood flow from both anterior cerebral arteries is included in the Doppler sample volume. Blood flow is away from the transducer in the ipsilateral (same side) ACA, and toward the transducer in the contralateral (opposite side) ACA.

During the ACA examination, sometimes it is possible to cross the midline and evaluate the contralateral ACA and MCA. Although this technique is not recommended for routine evaluation, it can be useful if a contralateral transtemporal window cannot be located.

Anterior Communicating Artery

The anterior communicating artery (ACoA) joins the two anterior cerebral arteries (A1 segments) at the midline. Doppler signals are usually obtained from the ACoA only when it is functioning as a collateral vessel. When there is balanced perfusion, and equal pressure, in each ACA, the ACoA is only a potential" collateral pathway and is "hemodynamically silent". Therefore it is not detectable by TCD. The ACoA Doppler signal is found at approximately 70-80 mm. If serving as a functional conduit, the direction of flow is away from the side supplying the blood, or conversely, toward the side supported by this collateral pathway. The ACoA becomes a channel that supplies both A2 ACA segments when one A1 ACA is artetic. This is a common anatomic variation and by itself should not be taken as a sign of internal carotid artery disease. With ICA obstructions, the ACoA is commonly being used as a collateral channel, and its Doppler signal at midline is characterized by its increased velocity and turbulence.

Terminal Internal Carotid Artery

At the completion of the ACA evaluation, the sample volume should be returned to the bi-directional reference signal, which is the terminal ICA bifurcation. The terminal ICA is examined by angling the transducer slightly inferiorly from the bifurcation. Since it is evaluated through the transtemporal window from an acute angle, blood flow is normally toward the transducer and has a low velocity signal (39 $\pm$ 9 cm/sec) (Figure 3-11). The ICA usually can be followed inferiorly for only a short distance.

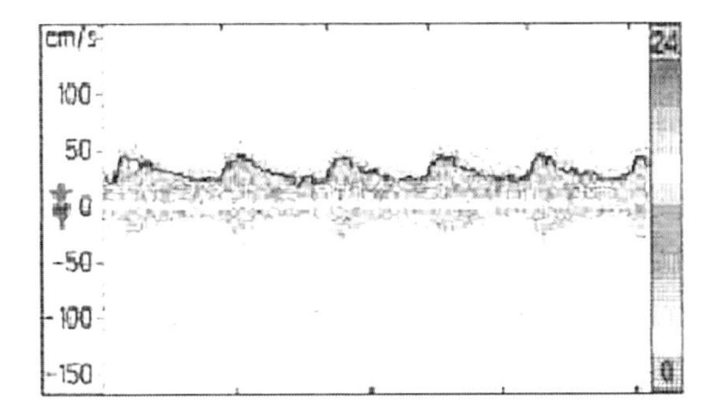

Figure 3-11. The terminal ICA Doppler signal. Depth of 64 mm; mean velocity is 32 cm/sec.

Posterior Cerebral Artery

Returning the sample volume to the reference signal at the t-ICA bifurcation, the posterior cerebral artery (PCA) is identified by angling the transducer posteriorly and slightly inferiorly, and by increasing the depth of the sample volume by 2-5 mm. Blood flow is normally toward the transducer in the proximal (P1) segment of the PCA, and the mean velocity is 39 $\pm$ 10 cm/sec (Figure 3-12). At each sample volume depth, it is important to adjust the angle of the transducer to obtain the best quality Doppler signal. The PCA mean velocity is usually lower than the MCA velocity, and the PCA is located deeper than 55 mm, which assists the operator in distinguishing it from the MCA. If a lower than expected velocity is obtained from the PCA, it may be due to insonation of the superior cerebellar artery which courses parallel to the posterior cerebral artery.

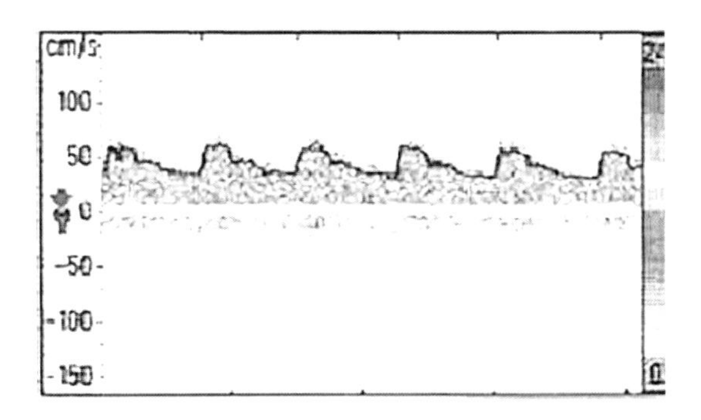

Figure 3-12. The PCA Doppler signal. Depth is 66 mm; mean velocity is 44 cm/sec.

The Doppler signal often becomes bi-directional as the sample volume approaches midline (70-80 mm) due to detection of flow in the ipsilateral PCA directed toward the transducer and blood flow away from the transducer in the contralateral PCA. If the operator has difficulty locating the PCA, returning to the terminal ICA bifurcation reference signal allows re-orientation of the transducer's angle.

The distal PCA (P2) segment is found in the range of 60-70 mm and is located by increasing the posterior angulation of the transducer from the P1 segment. Blood flow may be toward the transducer and change direction more distally. The P2 segment may produce a bi-directional signal due its tortuousity or branches. The P2 segment is difficult to routinely evaluate during nonimaging TCD examinations. The PCA Doppler signal may be confused with the superior cerebellar artery signal with a too posterior and caudal transducer angulation.

Another way to verify the insonation of the PCA was suggested by Aaslid.[13] He demonstrated an increase in PCA velocity of 16.4% in response to light stimuli, compared to only a 3.3% increase by the MCA. Although Aaslid's study was performed under controlled conditions, a PCA's Doppler signal can be monitored and evaluated for changes in velocity as the patient opens and closes her/his eyes. This may help in identifying the PCA when other identification criteria are not met.

Posterior Communicating Artery

Similar to the ACoA, the posterior communicating artery (PCoA) is identified only if it is functioning as a collateral pathway. When found, the PCoA Doppler signal has an increased velocity and is turbulent. The PCoA is located by angling the transducer posteriorly and slightly inferiorly from the terminal ICA bifurcation.

Common Carotid Artery Compression

Proper identification of the intracranial arteries is usually possible in most cases without common carotid artery (CCA) compression or vibration maneuvers. The effect of CCA compression or oscillations on the intracranial Doppler signals, however, may help in the identification of the intracranial arteries (MCA vs. PCA) or in assessing collateral pathways in special cases.

It is important to strongly emphasize that CCA compressions or oscillations are not routinely performed during a TCD examination. CCA compression or oscillation should be performed only by experienced personnel, and only if the CCA is disease free.

Carotid duplex imaging can determine the level of the CCA bifurcation and if any disease is present in the CCA. This is important because plaque dislodged by CCA compressions may cause thromboembolic complications.

Transorbital Window

The optic canal in the posterior orbit is the bony ostium, providing the ultrasound window for the transorbital approach. It allows access to the ophthalmic artery and the siphon of the internal carotid artery.

Since the ultrasound waves must transverse the eye, the examination time should be as short as possible and the acoustical intensity reduced to a low setting (10% of the maximum) to minimize ultrasound exposure. Although bioeffects on the eye have not been reported using current TCD equipment, it is prudent to exercise caution until evidence conclusively demonstrates safety.

It is suggested that patients remove contact lenses before the transorbital examination. If present, they may cause discomfort, and may scatter the ultrasound waves, thereby creating difficulty in locating the ultrasound window.

The TCD transducer is gently placed on the closed eyelid. Remember that with this approach, application of pressure is not needed if an ample amount of gel is used. If the operator is sitting at the head of the examination table, resting the hand on the patient's forehead will stabilize the operator's hand and avoids placing pressure on the closed eye. If the operator is standing on the side of the patient, the same stabilization may be accomplished by resting the operator's hand on the patient's cheek. Blinking is a natural response if the patient is not comfortable (Figure 3-13). Patients should be instructed to focus their eyes to the opposite side from that being examined. This will help divert the patient's attention and often reduces the artifact introduced by blinking. The transducer is aimed posteriorly and slightly medially toward the optic canal.

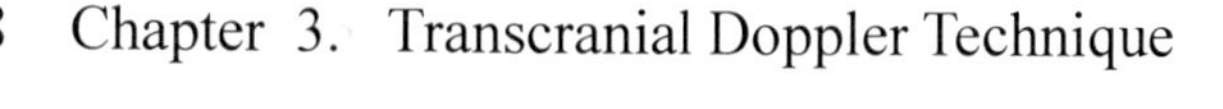

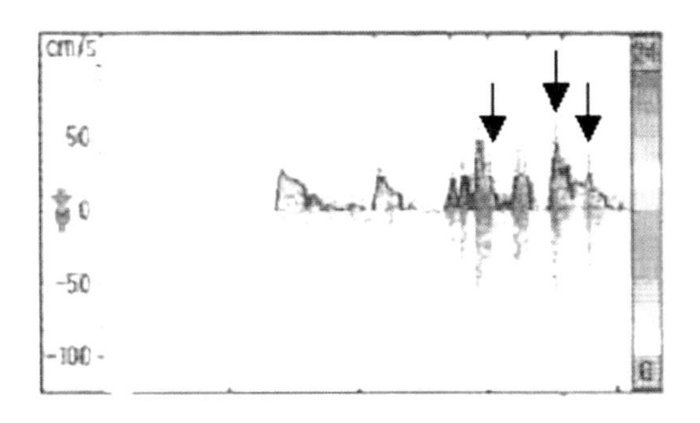

Figure 3-13. Artifact (arrows) in the ophthalmic artery Doppler signal due to blinking.

Ophthalmic Artery

The depth of the sample volume setting should be set at approximately 50 mm during the initial search for the ophthalmic artery (OA). The ultrasound beam is directed slightly medially along the anterior-posterior (sagittal) plane, and only small movements of the transducer along the surface of the eyelid are required. The ophthalmic artery is evaluated once the Doppler signal has been located and the signal optimized. The ophthalmic artery is usually found at depths ranging from 40-60 mm. Blood flow is normally directed toward the transducer and the mean velocity is 21 $\pm$ 5 cm/sec. (Figure 3-14). The OA Doppler signal has a pulsatility index higher than the intracranial arteries because it supplies orbital structures including muscles and it anastomoses with ECA arterial territories. The flow direction in the ophthalmic artery will be reversed when it is functioning as a collateral from the ECA branches because of severe disease of the ICA. Under these circumstances, the OA Doppler signal often takes on the waveform characteristics of a Doppler signal supplying a low resistance cerebral vascular bed.

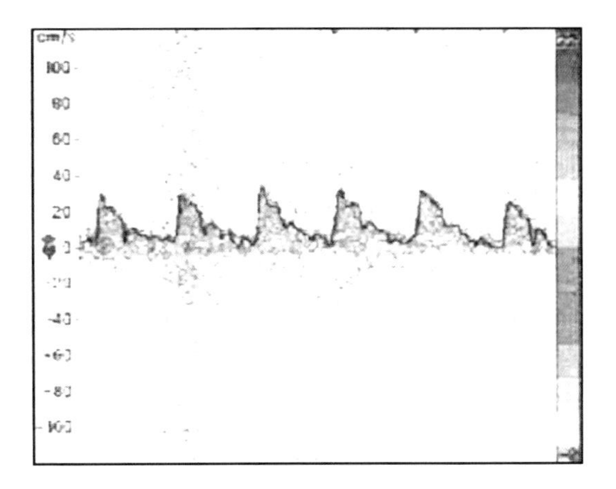

Figure 3-14. Ophthalmic artery Doppler signal. Depth of 46 mm; mean velocity is 16 cm/sec.

Carotid Siphon

After the ophthalmic artery has been evaluated, the depth of the sample volume is increased to examine the carotid siphon (CS). The carotid siphon is located at a depth of 60-80 mm and the mean velocity is 47 $\pm$ 14 cm/sec. A slight change in the transducer angle is often needed when making the transition from the ophthalmic artery to the carotid siphon. In addition, there is a change in the quality of the Doppler signal as the high pulsatility of the OA signal changes to the low pulsatility of the carotid siphon.

The specific sections of the carotid siphon (parasellar, genu, and supraclinoid) are sequentially examined, although all segments of the internal carotid siphon may not be identified during every examination. The segments of the siphon are distinguished by their direction of blood flow. The signal from the genu is bi-directional (Figure 3-15). Signals from the parasellar segment, which is proximal to the genu, can be located by angling the transducer inferiorly and blood flow is normally toward the transducer (Figure 3-16). The distal, supraclinoid portion of the carotid siphon is located by angling the transducer superiorly with blood flow normally away from the transducer (Figure 3-17). The bi-directional signal in the genu is an important landmark for the proper evaluation of the siphon segments. If signals from the proximal or distal carotid siphon cannot be located, the Doppler sample volume should be returned to the genu. Its characteristic waveform permits re-orientation of the transducer's angle to the internal carotid artery.

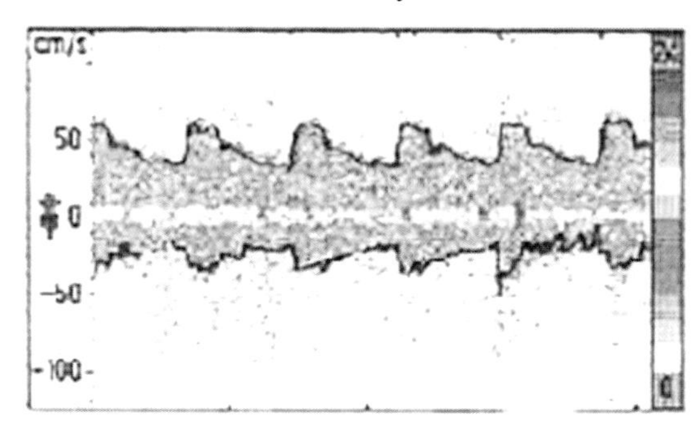

Figure 3-15. ICA genu Doppler signal at 66 mm demonstrating bi-directional blood flow.

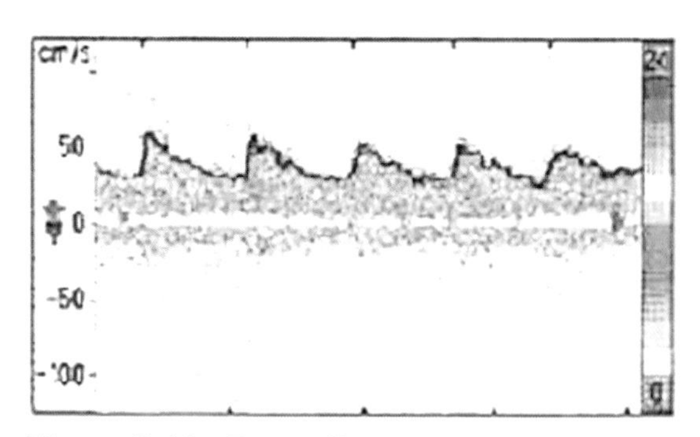

Figure 3-16. Parasellar segment of the ICA. Blood flow is toward the transducer and the mean velocity is 42 cm/sec.

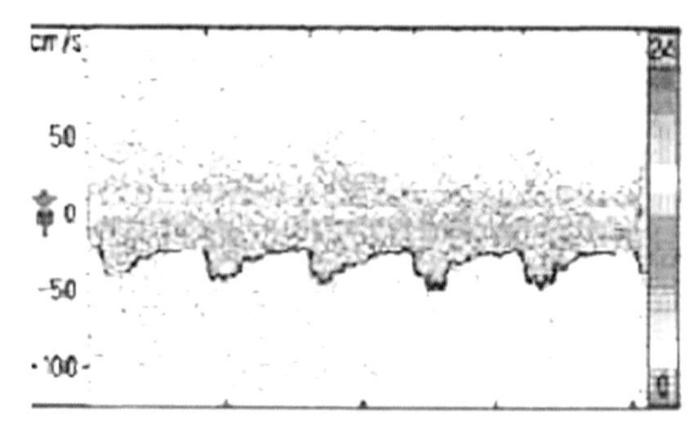

Figure 3-17. The supraclinoid segment of the ICA demonstrating blood flow away from the transducer.

Anterior Cerebral Artery (Contralateral)

Doppler signals from the contralateral anterior cerebral artery can be obtained from the transorbital approach. An oblique transorbital approach aiming the ultrasound beam superiorly and medially from the carotid siphon permits insonation of the anterior cerebral artery at depths approximately 70-80 mm. Blood flow in the contralateral ACA should be directed toward the transducer. This approach to the anterior cerebral arteries is technically difficult, is generally not recommended, but may be useful if a contralateral transtemporal window is absent.

Suboccipital Window

The evaluation of the intracranial vertebral arteries and the basilar artery is obtained by using the suboccipital approach. The foramen magnum is the large caudal ostium in the skull through which the spinal cord passes, and is the natural opening providing the suboccipital TCD window. Properly positioning the patient will make this approach much easier. If the patient's head is bowed slightly so the chin is toward the chest, the gap between the cranium and the atlas is increased, which considerably enlarges the suboccipital window. If the patient's head is bowed too much, however, the muscular anatomy of the suboccipital space makes locating the window more difficult.

The transducer is placed in the midline at the nape of the neck. In some patients, the transducer may need to be shifted slightly to either side to obtain good quality Doppler signals. The ultrasound beam should be aimed toward the bridge of the patient's nose. If a Doppler signal is not located from this approach, it is advisable to check for adequate transducer-gel contact prior to abandoning the examination. Additional acoustic gel is often necessary due to interference of the patient's hair with the transducer-gel contact.

Vertebral Artery

The search for the suboccipital window is performed with the sample volume depth setting in the range of 60-70 mm. A Doppler signal usually can be located if the transducer is aimed in the general direction of the bridge of the nose. A vertebral artery signal may be located by aiming the transducer slightly to either side of midline. The vertebral arteries can be evaluated by moving the transducer's angle laterally from side to side at each sample volume depth, or by tracing the vertebral artery one side at a time. The advantage of evaluating both vertebral arteries at each depth is that the operator is ensured that signals are obtained from the right and left sides by the transducer's angle and the relationship of one signal to the other.

The vertebral arteries are located in the depth range of 40-85 mm. Blood flow is normally away from the transducer toward the head and the mean velocity is 38 ± 10 cm (Figure 3-18). At each sample volume depth setting, the angle of the transducer should be adjusted to obtain the best quality Doppler signal. The vertebral artery's largest branch, the posterior inferior cerebellar artery (PICA), or other smaller branches may be included in the sample volume which might confound the signal by showing blood flow toward the transducer. Since the vertebral artery branches account for the bi-directional signals in this location, it is important to recognize this possibility and not misinterpret it as reversed blood flow in the vertebral artery. At more shallow depths, bi-directional signals are usually the result of tortuous vertebral arteries

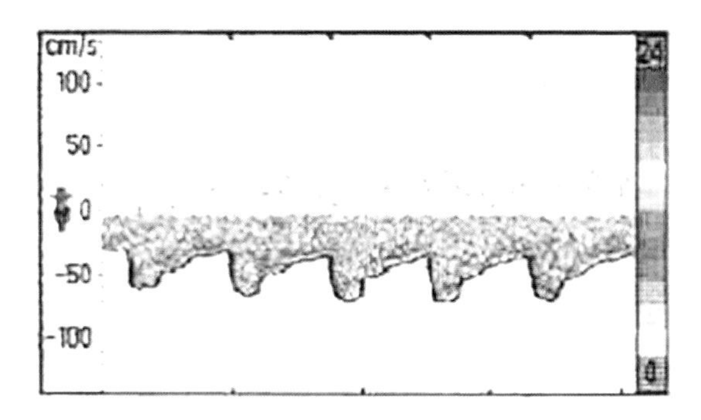

Figure 3-18. The vertebral artery Doppler signal. Depth of 66 mm; mean velocity is 40cm/sec.

Basilar Artery

Following the vertebral arteries distally by increasing the sample volume depth, occasionally a notable change can be demonstrated in the Doppler signal. This change in the Doppler signal indicates the origin of the basilar artery at the confluence of the vertebral arteries. In the basilar artery, blood flow continues to be away from the transducer and the mean velocity is 41 ± 10 cm/sec (Figure 3-19).

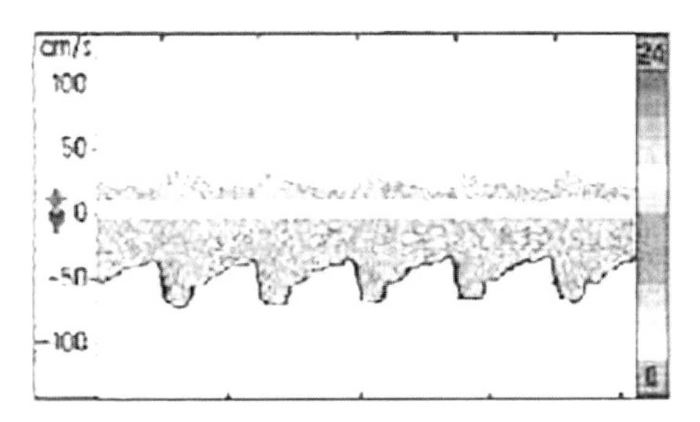

Figure 3-19. The basilar artery Doppler signal. Depth of 86 mm; mean velocity is 50 cm/sec.

The transducer's angle should be adjusted at each sample volume depth, and the intensity level increased to obtain the best quality Doppler signals as the basilar artery is traced. Differentiating the vertebral artery Doppler signal from the basilar artery signal may be difficult, because of natural anatomic variations. For example, if there is hypoplasia or occlusion of one vertebral artery, then separation of the remaining vertebral artery Doppler signal from the basilar artery signal may not be possible.

The basilar artery signal is usually located at depths greater than 80 mm, although the vertebral artery confluence may be deeper, requiring sample volume depth settings of 90-100 mm. Most basilar arteries are 2-3.5 cm in length. One reason for the variation in the depths of the arteries when evaluating the vertebrobasilar system is that the thickness of the suboccipital soft tissue is individually extremely variable. To evaluate the distal basilar artery, the transducer may need to be moved inferiorly on the neck and angled more superiorly.

Vertebral Artery Compression

Compression of the vertebral artery (VA) is helpful when trying to identify the branches of the posterior circulation. Although difficult, manual compression of the vertebral artery is possible by using finger pressure in the groove beneath the mastoid process. Considering the location of the vertebral artery within its bony canal, one can appreciate why complete compression is usually successful in only 50% of the cases. Since intense pressure is required to compress the vertebral artery, the best results are obtained if two examiners are involved - one operating the TCD equipment and the other performing the compression maneuver. Due to the amount of pressure needed to compress the vertebral arteries, patients' often complain of discomfort. Additionally, the operator must be careful in maintaining the position of the transducer. Compression of the ipsilateral VA will result in a diminished, obliterated or a reversed Doppler signal. The contralateral VAsignal should not change or may augment, and the basilar artery signal may not change or may decrease.

Submandibular Window

The submandibular window is used less frequently then the three approaches previously discussed. We use this approach routinely in patients with subarachnoid hemorrhage to obtain a Lindegaard ratio for grading spasm severity (see Chapter 6; Clinical Applications). The submandibular approach is an extension of the direct examination of the extracranial portion of the internal carotid artery and is used to examine the retromandibular and proximal intracranial portion of the internal carotid artery. Maintaining good transducer-gel contact is usually not a problem from the submandibular approach, unless the patient has a beard.

Internal Carotid Artery

To insonate the distal internal carotid artery, the transducer is placed at the angle of the mandible and aimed slightly medially pointed in a cephalad direction. The carotid canal is the ostium used during this TCD approach. The ICA can usually be tracked through its petrosal segment, and normally blood flow is away from the transducer (Figure 3-20). The depth of the sample volume varies depending on the ICA location and the amount of soft tissue present. The ICA is usually found at depths of 35-70 mm and the mean velocity is 37 ± 9 cm/sec. The operator must be careful to distinguish the ICA from the ECA when locating the Doppler signal from this approach (the ICA demonstrates a low resistance, and the ECA a high resistance). While examining the proximal portion of this segment of the ICA, venous Doppler signals may also be identified due to the simultaneous sampling of the adjacent internal jugular vein. A minor change in the transducer's angle often eliminates the venous Doppler signal.

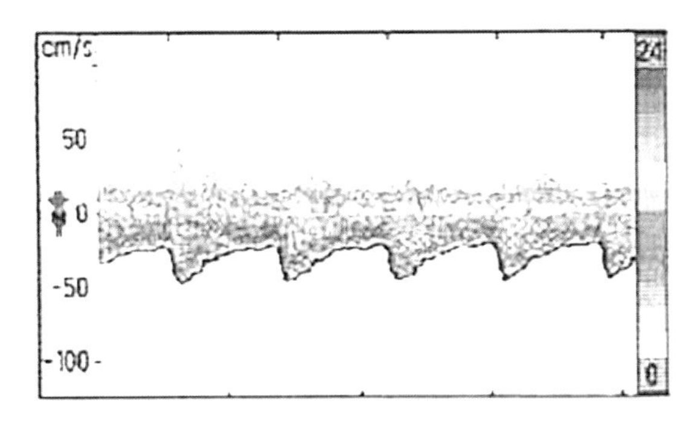

Figure 3-20. The internal carotid artery Doppler signal from the submandibular approach. Depth of 50mm; mean velocity is 32 cm/sec.

TCD Technique

A complete TCD examination incorporates the information obtained from the transtemporal, transorbital, submandibular approaches bilaterally, and from the suboccipital approach (Table 3-2).

Table 3-2. Depth and mean velocity ranges for the intracranial arteries in normal adults.

Artery	Depth (mm)	Mean velocity (cm/sec.)
MCA	30-67	62 ± 12
ACA (A1)	60-80	50 ±11
t-ICA	60-67	39 ± 9
PCA (p1)	55-80	39 ± 10
Ophthalmic	40-60	21 ± 5
Carotid siphon	60-80	47 ± 14
Vertebral	40-85	38 ± 10
Basilar	>80	41 ± 10
ICA (submandibular)	35-70	37 ± 9

The order of evaluating the windows, left/right side, or the intracranial arteries from each window may vary from institution to institution. The exact sequence of the steps in performing a TCD examination does not matter. However, it is beneficial to have a standard protocol adopted by each institution and have general examination guidelines (Table 3-3)

Table 3-3. TCD technical guidelines

- Obtain a patient history (focus on past medical history, risk factors, and symptoms)
- Be aware of the status of the patient's extracranial arteries
- Be familiar with intracranial arterial anatomy, physiology, and pathology
- Understand the equipment controls and how to adjust them
- Use stereo headphones to recognize subtle changes in the Doppler signals
- Use a large sample volume size (10-15mm)
- Adjust the transducer at each depth setting to obtain the best quality Doppler signal
- Compare the Doppler spectral waveforms from the anterior and posterior circulation, and from the right and left sides
- Notice the Doppler spectral waveform configuration
- Establish institutional technical protocols and diagnostic criteria for the various clinical applications
- Perform routine quality assurance

The examination of the intracranial arteries is not always technically successful, either due to inability in locating a TCD window or failure to identify specific intracranial arteries. The operator must be confident in her/his technical ability, be aware of the technique's limitations (Table 3-4), and be flexible in her/his technique making the necessary adjustments to achieve a complete, good quality, and reproducible examination in each patient (Table 3-5).

Table 3-4. Technical limitations of TCD

• Operator experience
• Absent/Poor transtemporal window
• Improper equipment settings
• Improper angle of the transducer
• Patient movement
• Anatomic variation
• Arterial misidentification

The Pediatric Patient

The TCD examination may be performed in the pediatric patient.[14,15] Clinical applications in this population are to assess patients with: sickle cell disease, Moyamoya disease, premature atherosclerosis, stroke, arterial dissection, vasospasm, and various cardiac abnormalities.

When performing TCD examinations in children, the operator should be aware of several changes in technique that will improve the quality of the examination in this specific population. Before beginning the TCD examination, the test should be explained to the child. To reduce fear and anxiety, allowing the child to touch the gel, listen to the Doppler signals, and observe the transducer being used on someone else will improve the child's cooperation.

Prior to beginning the examination it is necessary to measure the child's head. As children grow and their heads become larger, the bitemporal measurement is necessary to define the depth of the patient's midline (half the bitemporal measurement). This measurement is critical to accurately perform a TCD examination in a child, because with large transtemporal windows, it is easy to move across midline and evaluate the contralateral arteries by error. In addition, the expected depth range for the intracranial arteries will vary as the child's head diameter increases.

The four TCD ultrasound windows may be used when performing an examination in a child. The TCD windows are usually large and easy to locate in most children. Because of the large windows, the TCD power/intensity control setting should be reduced. The power/intensity level should be set at a maximum, however, if it is difficult to locate the transtemporal window. Additionally, many children will not tolerate the ultrasound evaluation via the transorbital window. If using this window is necessary in a child, this approach should be performed last. When using the transorbital window, the operator is reminded to decrease the Doppler output/intensity level to a minimum.

A technical challenge when performing TCD examinations in children is that they often will only lie still for a short time. In some cases, allowing the child to move between the evaluations of the different windows may be beneficial and will improve the quality of the overall examination. If a child will not lie still or is afraid, the examination may be performed with the child sitting in their caregiver's lap. Although this patient position is not ideal, it is possible to complete the examination with the child in this position. The operator must pay special attention to maintaining proper transducer-to-arteryangle when performing the test when the child is in this position.

Additionally, when performing TCD in children, a smaller sample volume size (6 mm) will usually provide good quality Doppler signals. Using a smaller sample volume size will also be useful when trying to isolate the small intracranial arteries.

The operator should also document if the child is crying or falls asleep during the examination, because this will change the patient's cerebral blood flow, and have an affect on the intracranial arterial velocities recorded. If possible, try to reschedule the examination. If the examination must be performed, wake the sleeping patient, or take the time to calm the patient who is afraid.

Intracranial arterial velocities are increased in children compared to adults. For example, in a child who is 10 year old, the mean velocity in the middle cerebral artery is approximately 95 cm/sec. To accurately measure the increased velocities obtained when examining children, the velocity scale needs to be increased or the zero baseline should be lowered to accurately display the spectral Doppler waveform.

Although the TCD examination in children can be challenging for the TCD operator, it can also be a lot of fun and very rewarding.

Table 3-5. Technical hints for performing TCD examinations

Challenge	Action
No Doppler Signal Absent window, window not located, poor patient positioning, or an occluded intracranial artery	1) Undergo a systematic search for a window. A window may be located by repositioning the transducer on the skin, changing the angle of the transducer, or by changing the depth of the sample volume. 2) Check the equipment control settings to ensure that the maximum power is being used especially when using the transtemporal window. Adjusting the gain setting may also prove to be valuable when searching for a window. 3) Add more ultrasound gel to maintain good transducer-to-skin contact. 4) Use a 1 MHz transducer for patients with thick temporal bones. 5) Reposition the patient to help in locating a Doppler signal, especially from the suboccipital window. 6) Use headphones to eliminate extraneous noise so that subtle Doppler signals may be detected.
Poor quality Doppler signal Small or poor window, improper equipment control settings, poor technique, poor patient positioning, or intracranial pathology.	1. Perform steps 1-6 (listed above). 2. Document any changes in blood flow velocity or spectral Doppler waveform shape that may indicate intracranial pathology
Multiple Doppler signals Large sample volume size, anatomic variation, or overlapping vessels.	1) Try using a smaller sample volume size. 2) Search for a better window by repositioning the transducer on the skin or by changing the angle of the transducer.
Background noise in Doppler signal Improper gain settings or placement of sample volume.	1) Adjust the gain setting so that the Doppler spectral waveform is optimized and the background noise is minimized. 2) Carefully adjust the angle of insonation to improve the signal-to-noise ratio. 3) Change the sample volume depth setting by a small increment to improve the quality of the signal.

Table 3-5, (continued). Technical hints for performing TCD examinations

Challenge	Action
Artifact in Doppler signal Patient movement, transducer movement, inadequate amount of ultrasound gel.	1) Take the time to put the patient at ease or answer any questions. 2) Minimize transducer movement by properly adjusting the operator's position (arm resting on examination table). 3) Adjust the gain setting so that the Doppler spectral waveform is optimized and the background noise is minimized. 4) Carefully adjust the angle of insonation to improve the signal-to-noise ratio. 5) Change the sample volume depth setting by a small increment to improve the quality of the signal.
Aliasing of Doppler signal Detected frequency exceeding the Nyquist limit.	1) Increase the PRF setting. 2) Decrease the zero baseline to increase the velocity scale in one direction.
" I am lost !" Not following examination protocol, patient movement, unusual window, anatomic variations, or intracranial pathology.	1) Undergo a systematic search for a better window. A window may be located by repositioning the transducer on the skin, changing the angle of the transducer, or by changing the depth of the sample volume. If an unusual window is used, check the angle of the transducer. 2) Locate the landmark t-ICA bifurcation signal and use it to locate the other arteries when using the transtemporal approach. 3) Follow the examination protocol, ultrasonically "tracing" each intracranial artery. 4) Remember that the patient's physiologic factors and any disease of the extracranial vessels may have an effect on the intracranial Doppler spectral waveforms (velocity and configuration). 5) Take the time to put the patient at ease or answer any questions. 6) Remember the limitations of the technique.

References

1. Aaslid R, Markwalder T-M, Nornes H. Noninvasive transcranial Doppler ultrasound recording of flow velocity in basal cerebral arteries. J Neurosurg 1982; 57:769-774.

2. Kloetzsch C, Popescu O, Berlit P. A new 1-MHz-probe for transcranial Doppler sonography in patients with inadequate temporal bone windows. Ultrasound Med Biol 1998;24:101-103.

3. Georgiadis D, Karatschai R, Uhlmann F, Lindner A. Diagnostic yield of a 1-MHz transducer in evaluation of the basal cerebral arteries. J Neuroimaging 1999;9:15-18.

4. Moehring M, Spencer MP. Power M-mode Doppler (PMD) for observing cerebral blood flow and tracking emboli. Ultrasound Med Biol. 2002; 28(1):49-57.

5. Alexandrov AV, Demchuk AM, Burgin WS. Insonation method and diagnostic flow signatures for transcranial power motion (M-mode) Doppler. J Neuroimaging 2002; 12:236-244.

6. Aaslid R. Transcranial Doppler Examination Techniques. Chapter 4. In: Aaslid R (Ed), Transcranial Doppler Sonography, New York, Springer-Verlag, 1986:39-59.

7. Sound Ergonomics LLC. Consultants for Sonographer Health. Accessed on December 5, 2001. http:/ soundergonomics.com

8. Grolimund P. Transmission of ultrasound through the temporal bone. Chapter 2. In: Aaslid R (Ed), Transcranial Doppler Sonography, New York:Springer-Verlag,1986:10-21.

9. Eden A. Letter to the Editor. Effect of emitted power on waveform intensity in transcranial Doppler. Stroke 1991; 22:533.

10. Halsey JH. Letter to the Editor. Stroke 1991;22:533-534.

11. Gomez CR, Gomez SM, Hall IS. The elusive transtemporal window: a technical and demographic study. J Cardiovasc Technol 1989;8:171-172.

12. Marinoni M, Ginanneschi A, Forleo P, Amaducci L. Technical limits in transcranial Doppler recording: Inadequate acoustic windows. Ultrasound Med Biol 1997;23:1275-1277.

13. Aaslid, R. Visually evoked dynamic blood flow response of the human cerebral circulation. Stroke 1987; 18:771-775.

14. Bode H. Pediatric applications of transcranial Doppler sonography. New York:Springer-Verlag, 1988.

15. Hirsch W, Hiebsch W, Teichler H, Schluter A. Transcranial Doppler sonography in children: review of a seven-year experience. Clin Radiol 2002;57:492-497.

Chapter 4
Transcranial Color Doppler Imaging

Color Doppler imaging is currently being used to investigate the intracranial arterial circulation. To obtain consistently reliable studies with transcranial color Doppler imaging (TCDI), the operator must appreciate the importance of proper patient positioning, use the available anatomic landmarks that are important for the accurate identification of the intracranial arteries, and be knowledgeable of the proper use of the instrument controls. The examination time may be shortened and its accuracy may increase by using the gray scale image and the color display to guide the transcranial Doppler evaluation.

This chapter describes: 1) the suggestions for instrument control settings, 2) TCDI techniques, and 3) the potential advantages and limitations of using TCDI.

Equipment. Instrument controls and control settings vary depending on the manufacturer of the color Doppler imaging system. Therefore, it is important for the operator to be familiar with her/his imaging system. The following discussion of instrumentation is generic to all state-of-the-art ultrasound imaging systems. Hard copy records of the spectral waveforms may be made using any of the standard formats, but a videocassette recording has the advantage of capturing the audio signal in addition to the Doppler spectral waveforms.

TCDI is performed with a phased array imaging transducer. A 2 MHz transducer (imaging and Doppler) is ideal for this application. However, transmitting frequencies as high as 3.5 MHz have been used with varying success.

High quality TCDI depends upon the proper adjustment of several instrument controls. It is important to optimize the gray scale image, know how each color control will independently affect the image, and understand how the different controls affect each other.[1] Appropriate adjustment of specific controls may be defined by the patient's arterial hemodynamics and the information that is relevant to the patient being evaluated.

Gray scale image. The gray scale image is produced by back-scatter echoes that originate along sound wave propagation through tissue interfaces. The received sound waves are amplified, converted, and mapped to an imaging process curve that relates echo intensity to a shade of gray. The stronger the echo received by the transducer, the brighter the shade of gray. This is often referred to as brightness mode, or B-mode imaging. Depending upon the timing of the echoes received, it is arranged along a line within the image corresponding to its appropriate depth.

Gain. Image gain adjusts the degree of amplification to received echoes, independent of depth. Gain, however, can be selectively adjusted at certain depths by the times gain compensation (TGC) control. To be able to selectively compensate for the differences in received reflection due to reflector depth is important because the amplitude and intensity of the sound waves decrease as they travel through tissue. Additionally, adjusting the image gain to the proper levels is important because it affects the appearance of the color Doppler display. The image gain may need to be adjusted during a TCDI examination.

Focal zone. The depth range at which the focus of the ultrasound beam is optimal is called the focal zone. Image quality, color resolution, and Doppler sensitivity are maximized in the focal zone. The focal zone is varied depending on the area of interest in the image. If the focal zone cannot be adjusted to the exact area of interest, it is customary to place it slightly deeper to achieve the best quality image.

Frame rate. The frequency (Hz) with which the image display is updated with new image data (image frames per second) is called the image frame rate. A fast frame rate ensures good temporal resolution and thus there is accurate depiction of motion and the rapid hemodynamics associated with intracranial blood flow. Frame rate decreases with increases in the image depth, the image width, and with multiple focuses.

Image sector width. The sector width of the gray scale image can be adjusted on most instruments. A smaller width reduces the volume of tissue studied, thereby decreasing the amount of gray scale information processed for a given frame. Less gray scale information, with the color Doppler data remaining the same, increases the frame rate. Using a small sector width does not compromise transcranial color Doppler imaging since the entire circle of Willis usually can be evaluated with a narrow setting. If necessary, the anterior and posterior circulations can be evaluated separately by changing the angle of the transducer, by changing the position of the color box, or by steering the image sector.

Dynamic range. Compression of the gray scale information to a usable display range is termed the dynamic range. It permits the operator to highlight the part of the gray scale that is of interest. The higher the dynamic range, the larger the range of gray scale values that enhance tissue texture. During TCDI, a dynamic range of 45-50 dB creates a visually pleasing image.

COLOR DOPPLER

Color box/overlay. In most duplex imaging systems, the colors are displayed in a small area designated the color "box". The color box can be moved to the area of interest on the gray scale image to investigate blood flow. Steering the color box changes the incidence angle and may improve the color display. The size of the color box is controllable by the operator. Since the image frame rate decreases with increasing width, it is important to keep the color box as small as possible. During TCDI, the entire circle of Willis can often be captured within a small color box. If not, to maintain a good frame rate, the color box should remain small, and the anterior and posterior circulations should be evaluated separately by moving the position of the color box.

Color map/bar/wheel. The color bar represents the range of frequencies or calculated velocities that are obtainable at a designated pulse repetition frequency (PRF). The color baseline, displayed in black, represents zero and divides the color bar into maximum positive (toward the transducer) and negative (away from the transducer) velocities (Figure 4-1). The velocities are displayed as dark shades of color changing to lighter shades as the calculated velocity values increase.

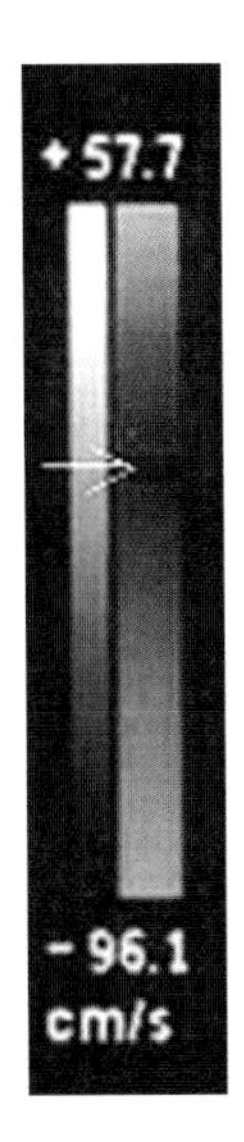

Figure 4-1. The color bar display. Positive Doppler shifts are displayed in red and negative Doppler shifts are displayed in blue. The arrow points to the black zero baseline.

Directional changes are seen in the color display as the darkest shade of one color adjacent to the darkest shade of the other color going through the zero baseline (black). The generic color assignment in vascular ultrasound examinations is red for arteries and blue for veins. The color assignment used during TCDI, however, represents blood flow direction in the intracranial arteries relative to the transducer. Red is assigned to blood flow toward the transducer and is displayed above the baseline. Shades of blue represent blood flow away from the transducer and are displayed below the baseline. *The color orientation should never be changed during a TCDI examination.* The operator must take care to avoid inverting the color assignment orientation, and the interpreter must be cautious when reviewing the intracranial images.

Wall filter. The color wall filter is a high-pass filter that permits higher frequencies to be displayed and allows the operator to selectively remove low frequencies due to motion artifact. On many instruments, the wall filter is directly connected to the color PRF and will automatically increase as the PRF is increased. Increasing the color wall filter will increase the length of the black zero baseline in the color bar. It is recommended to use the lowest wall filter that can be achieved in order to visualize the most discriminating blood flow patterns. The color wall filter should initially be set at 100 Hz for TCDI.

Gain. The color gain control adjusts amplification of the displayed color signal. The color gain is set high for TCDI, and requires adjusting during the examination to accommodate changing signal strengths (Figure 4-2 A, B, C). If the color gain is too low, intracranial blood flow may not be detected. On the other hand, if the color gain is set too high, random color data ("noise") is introduced into the display. The best method of adjusting color gain is to increase it to "over gain", and then decrease it until the random color data disappears from the surrounding brain parenchyma.

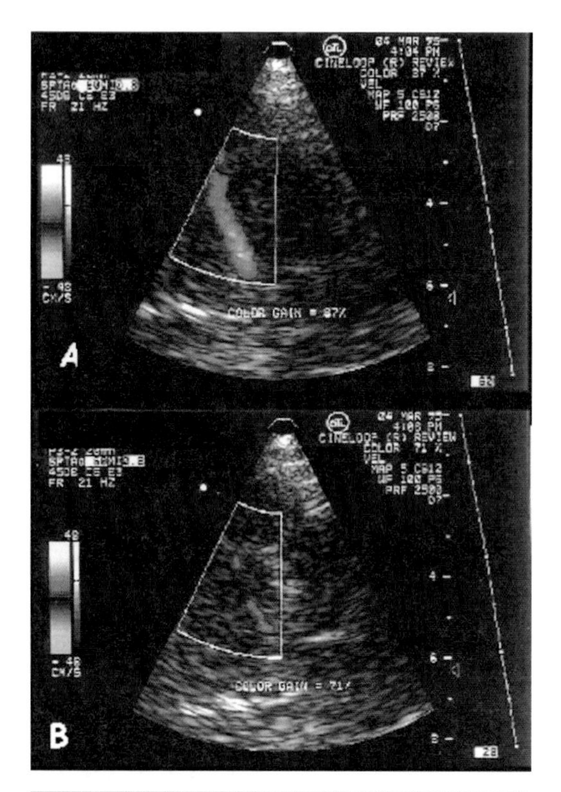

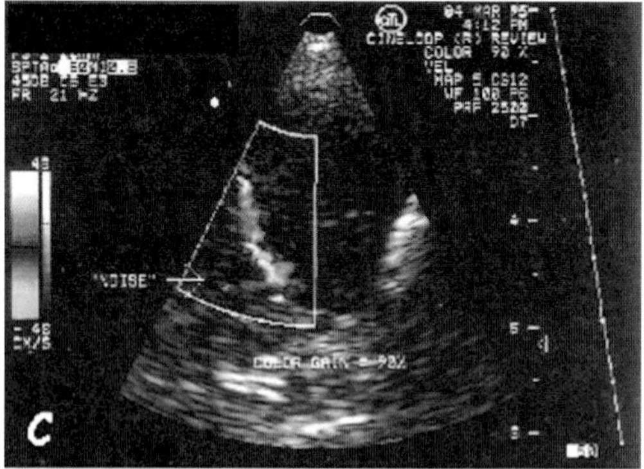

Figure 4-2. The middle cerebral artery with three different color gain settings. A) Proper gain setting, B) Decreased gain setting, and C) Increased gain setting.

Pulse repetition frequency. The number of ultrasound pulses emitted by the transducer per second is called the pulse repetition frequency (PRF). The PRF is adjustable and is limited by the depth of the image. Decreasing the image depth increases the PRF. The velocity values on the color bar are calculated using a standard angle, which is usually zero degrees. Since most of the vessels examined do not lie parallel to the ultrasound scan line (i.e. a 0 degree angle), the color velocity values should be considered as qualitative information. The upper limit of the Doppler shift that can be detected by pulsed Doppler instruments is equal to one half of the PRF, which is termed the Nyquist limit. Aliasing occurs if the Nyquist limit is exceeded.

The color PRF may need to be adjusted throughout the TCDI examination to accommodate the constantly changing velocity patterns that are often present in intracranial arterial cerebral blood flow. The color PRF should initially be set at 2500-3000 Hz for TCDI. If the PRF is set too high, the lower velocities may not be detected on the color display. If the PRF is set too low, aliasing occurs which may be misinterpreted as turbulence or reversed blood flow direction (Figure 4-3).

The color PRF may require adjusting when using one TCDI window compared to another, when trying to locate one artery from another within the same window, and when evaluating the anterior circulation from the posterior circulation, from the transtemporal approach. The PRF needs to be increased in a stenosis, and decreased to visualize post-stenotic turbulence, bruits, and to detect low cerebral blood flow states.

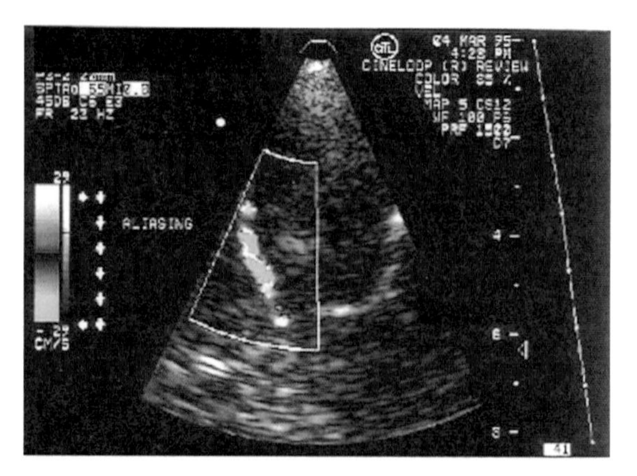

Figure 4-3. The middle cerebral artery with a decreased color PRF setting (aliasing).

Aliasing. Aliasing occurs with all pulsed Doppler systems and is observed when the detected frequency exceeds the Nyquist limit (one half the PRF). This increase in frequency may be due to a narrowing of the vessel, but can also be due to a decrease in Doppler angle. Color Doppler imaging displays aliasing as "wrapping around" the color bar. The aliased frequencies are displayed as the lightest shade of one color adjacent to the lightest shade of the opposite color on the color bar.

Increasing the PRF, adjusting the color baseline to increase the PRF in the appropriate direction, or decreasing the image depth, which results in an increased PRF, can eliminate aliasing. During TCDI, it is best to increase the color PRF to eliminate aliasing.

Ensemble length. The ensemble length, or color sensitivity, is the number of pulse cycles per scan line from which the color frequency information is derived. On many instruments, the manufacturer presets this feature. The higher the number, the more robust the color displayed. Increasing the color sensitivity sends more pulses down each line; therefore, it will take longer to create one frame (decreased frame rate). Decreasing the color box width to compensate preserves the image frame rate. The greater the ensemble length, the more reliable the color information will be in representing low velocity information.

Persistence. Specialized frame averaging allowing color to remain ("persist") from frame to frame is termed persistence, which gives the appearance of increased color sensitivity and "filling" of the vessel (smoother image). As one increases persistence, there will be a concomitant decrease in the frame rate, and an increase in temporal averaging. An increase in color persistence is advantageous in detecting very slow blood flow, and if the persistence is adjusted too high, it may mask rapid hemodynamic changes. If one wishes to evaluate changes in vascular resistance, i.e. monitoring cerebral circulatory arrest (brain death), persistence should be turned off to allow differentiation of systolic and diastolic flow.

Priority. When both color and gray scale are being acquired and displayed simultaneously, the echo-write priority control allows the operator to select whether the instrument will write color or echo information. A threshold is assigned on the gray scale bar below in which color will be preferentially displayed in place of echo information. Although this control is not adjustable on some duplex imaging systems, the same effect is obtained by adjusting the image gain or time gains compensation control for the gray scale. Since intracranial arteries are small, and reliable visualization of the vessel wall is not currently feasible, the hemodynamic details of blood flow have superseded in importance the anatomic details on the gray scale image. It is important to adjust the color priority high, allowing color to be written wherever there is blood flow. If the threshold is set too low, or if the gray scale image gain is too high, blood flow may not be visualized.

Power. The power Doppler display involves the encoding of the strength (intensity, amplitude) of the Doppler shifts with colors based on a selected power map. Values are assigned to the Doppler shift amplitudes (concentration of the moving blood cells) instead of the Doppler shift frequencies. This type of imaging is less angle dependent, free of aliasing, and demonstrates an increased sensitivity to slow flow and blood flow in deep and small vessels. The disadvantages of power imaging are the loss of blood flow direction, speed, and the character of the flow.

Doppler spectral waveforms

Doppler. Detection of intracranial blood flow is obtained using a pulsed-wave Doppler. The real time display of all Doppler shift frequencies over time is the Doppler spectral waveform. Time (seconds) is recorded along the horizontal axis, and velocity (frequency) is on the vertical axis. Velocity is recorded in centimeters per second (cm/sec). The Doppler scale is divided by a zero baseline; with a positive shift (toward the transducer) displayed above the baseline, and a negative Doppler shift (away from the transducer) below the baseline. Accurate recording of the intracranial Doppler spectral waveforms is critical, since this is the basis for interpretation of the TCDI examination (Figure 4-4). At each sample volume depth the transducer should be angled to obtain the best quality Doppler signal. This usually takes time and the operator should not settle for the first signal located.

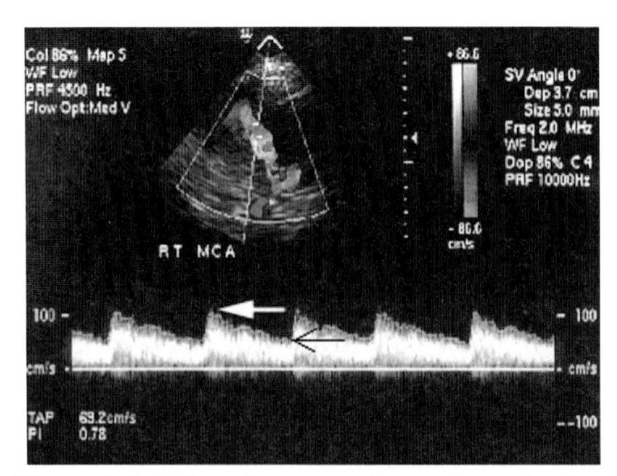

Figure 4-4. A Doppler spectral waveform obtained from the middle cerebral artery. Peak systolic velocity is 100 cm/sec (white arrow), end diastolic velocity is 52 cm/sec (black arrow), mean velocity is 69 cm/sec, and the pulsatility index is 0.78.

The Doppler spectral waveforms recorded during a TCDI examination are similar to those obtained from the cervical (ICA). Diastolic flow is present throughout the cardiac cycle because of the low peripheral resistance of the brain. Describing the spectral waveforms from the intracranial arteries; peak velocity refers to the highest velocity noted in systole, and end diastolic velocity is the maximal velocity just prior to the acceleration phase (systole) of the next waveform. During TCDI examinations, however, mean velocity is the parameter reported. The preference to use mean velocity instead of peak velocity for TCDI examinations is because the mean velocity is less affected by systemic factors such as heart rate, contractility, total peripheral resistance, and correlates better with perfusion.[2]

The mean velocity calculated by TCDI equipment is based upon the time average of the outline velocity (maximum velocity envelope). The velocity envelope is a trace of the peak velocities as a function of time. The quality of the maximum velocity envelope is responsible for the accuracy of the instrument's calculation of the mean velocity and the pulsatility index (P.I.). The operator adjusts the Doppler gain and intensity levels to obtain the best signal-to-noise ratio. Improper gain adjustment or intensity settings result in unsatisfactory maximum velocity envelopes. If this occurs, the automatic calculations produced by the TCDI equipment are invalid. The mean velocity can be estimated in these cases, however, by manually tracing the Doppler waveforms with the instrument controls or by positioning the horizontal cursor at the velocity where the area below the peak velocity and above the cursor are equal to the area below the cursor and above the peak velocity envelope in diastole.

Another method to estimate the mean velocity of a TCDI signal is to use one of the following two formulas:

$$\frac{\text{(peak systolic - end diastolic)} + \text{end diastolic}}{3}$$

or

$$\frac{\text{peak systolic} + \text{(end diastolic x 2)}}{3}$$

Depending upon the manufacturing company, the maximum velocity envelope on TCDI equipment may only be functional above the zero baseline. The values calculated with each display sweep apply only to the Doppler spectral waveform that appears above the baseline. If blood flow is away from the transducer (below the baseline), it may be necessary to change the direction of the waveform on the display to above the baseline so that the equipment can perform the computations. It is important that the operator and interpreter be aware of the direction icon on the display that indicates whether blood flow is away from or toward the transducer.

Sample volume size. The sample volume is the specific area interrogated along the ultrasound beam. Blood flowing within the sample volume generates the velocities detected by the Doppler equipment. During a TCDI evaluation, the depth of the sample volume varies as the different intracranial arteries are evaluated. Changes in sample volume depth on imaging systems may result in a change in the pulse repetition frequency (PRF). The sample volume size usually should be from 10 to 15 mm for the best signal-to-noise ratio.

Using a large Doppler sample volume size to evaluate the small intracranial arteries causes two effects on the spectral Doppler waveform. First, the sample volume size is larger than the diameter of any intracranial artery. Thus, the Doppler shift will contain the fast moving blood flow from the center of the vessel's lumen and the slow moving blood flow along the walls of the artery. Because the sample volume includes the blood flow from the entire lumen of the artery, all TCDI Doppler spectral waveforms will demonstrate spectral broadening. Thus, spectral broadening is not used as an interpretation criterion for TCDI examinations. Second, the large sample volume size usually contains Doppler frequency shifts from more than one artery or from one artery and its branches. This may be displayed in the Doppler spectral waveform as blood flowing in both directions (toward and away from the transducer) or a Doppler signal from one artery with a more intense signal from a second artery displayed within the first artery's signal.

Angle. TCDI is performed assuming a zero degree angle. Although angle adjusted (corrected) velocities may be used during imaging, it is not recommended. Assuming a zero degree angle, the intracranial arterial velocities acquired with transcranial color Doppler imaging should be similar to the nonimaging technique. If adjusted velocities are desired, the operator must adjust to the color display because the walls of the intracranial arteries cannot be visualized during imaging. Angle adjusted velocities will be higher than the velocities recorded assuming a zero degree angle (Figure 4-5).

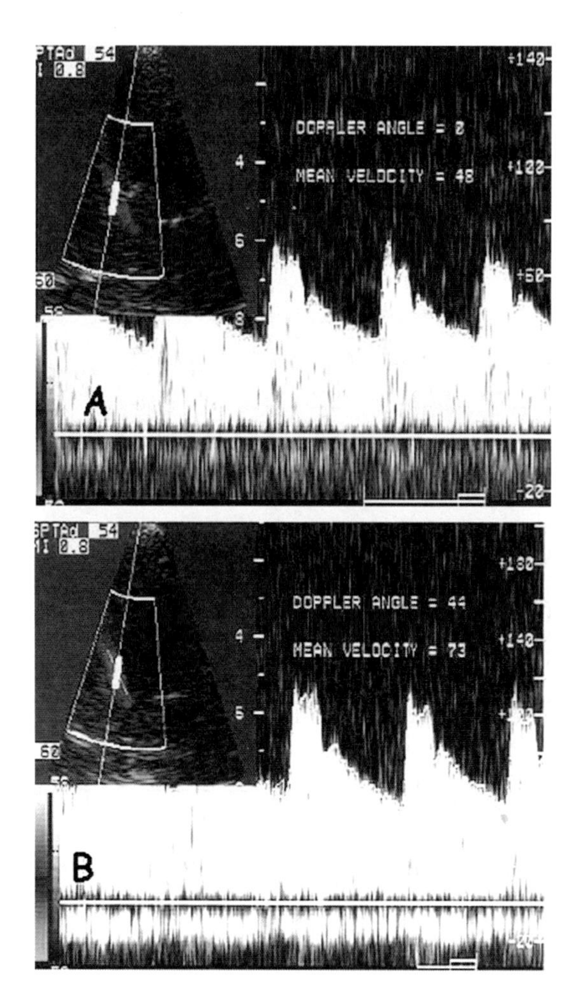

Figure 4-5. The MCA Doppler signal obtained with A) a zero degree angle (mean velocity is 48 cm/sec.), and B) angle adjustment (mean velocity is 73 cm/sec.).

Wall filter. The wall filter eliminates motion artifact. This is usually not a problem with performing a TCDI examination. Therefore, a low wall filter up to 100 Hz is suggested. The operator can usually select the wall filter, but on some instruments, it may vary depending on the PRF.

Gain. The Doppler gain serves as an amplifier for the incoming Doppler signals. During a TCDI study, it is important to adjust the Doppler gain so that the peak trace envelope, which is instrument dependent, accurately follows the spectral Doppler waveform. Occasionally, amplification of weak Doppler signals produces considerable background noise, the peak trace envelope is inaccurate, and the operator has to calculate the mean velocity.

Pulse repetition frequency (PRF). The number of ultrasound pulses emitted by the transducer per second is the pulse repetition frequency (PRF). The PRF for the Doppler spectral waveform display is independent of the PRF setting for the color Doppler display. Higher Doppler shifts will be detected with a higher PRF, but this also increases the chance of range ambiguity artifact. The upper limit to Doppler shifts that can be detected is one half the PRF, the Nyquist limit. When the Nyquist limit is exceeded, aliasing occurs in the Doppler spectral waveform display. To display increased velocities (eliminate aliasing), the operator can increase the velocity scale and/or decrease the zero baseline to increase the scale in one direction.

Output. Safety issues concerning ultrasound that include thermal and the cavitational bioeffect mechanism are related to Doppler output (intensity). The operator adjusts this control, and the values that measure this potential problem are displayed differently by the various manufacturers (i.e. spatial peak-temporal average [SPTA], percentage [%], mechanical index [MI], etc.). During TCDI, the Doppler power should be increased for adequate penetration, except when using the transorbital window when the Doppler output should be decreased. The Doppler output should be at the lowest level necessary and applied for the shortest duration possible to obtain good clinical information. The ALARA ("as low as reasonably achievable") principle should be applied during TCDI.

Position

Patient.

TCDI examinations are performed with the patient in the supine position. An examination table is preferable, however, if the patient is immobile, s/he can be examined lying on a stretcher or in a hospital bed. The patient's neck should be straight with their head placed on a small pillow. Maintaining patient comfort cannot be overemphasized, since head movements are minimized which may change the transducer-artery angle. Respiratory changes due to anxiety are also reduced thereby avoiding hypercapnia or hypocapnia, which cause fluctuations in cerebral blood flow. Before beginning the examination, enough time should be allowed for the stabilization of the patient's heart rate and blood pressure.

The supine position allows access to the transtemporal, transorbital, and submandibular windows, whereas other positions are used for the suboccipital approach. The suboccipital examination can be performed with the patient lying supine and the head turned to one side, with the patient sitting and the head lowered slightly towards their chest, or with the patient lying on the side with the head bowed slightly so the chin touches their chest. We have found the suboccipital examination easier if the patient is able to tolerate lying on their side.

Operator.

A good quality TCDI examination requires concentration; therefore, the operator should not be rushed or interrupted. Time, patience, and alert thinking are required for consistently accurate TCDI examinations. The operator should be schooled in Doppler ultrasound principles, cerebrovascular hemodynamics, and intracranial anatomy, as well as appreciate the potential intracranial collateral blood flow patterns.

The operator sits near the patient's head and stabilizes the examining arm by resting the elbow on the examination table. This placement of the arm eliminates minor spontaneous hand movements that may cause intracranial arterial Doppler signals to be lost, and prevents motion artifact from being introduced into the signal. From this position, the operator also has equal access to both sides of the patient's head, permitting the best orientation of the transducer to the body.

It is critical that the operator maintains a comfortable and ergonomically sound position when performing TCDI examinations.[3] Proper body mechanics and postural alignment will assist in avoiding pain and injury. It is important to have an easily adjustable examination table for the patient and an adjustable chair or stool for the operator. In addition, it is very important to support your arm when scanning, placing a pillow underneath your arm if necessary. Use a relaxed grip on the transducer. Remember that it is critical to your health to take a few minutes to find the proper position.

During bedside examinations, it is advantageous for the operator to position herself/himself behind the head of the bed. In some instances (i.e. intensive care units), it may be difficult for the operator to achieve this position. Whatever extra effort is exerted for proper positioning will be rewarded by improved results and will be helpful in minimizing unhealthy body positions. The optimal second choice is to stand on either side of the patient, resting the examining arm on the bed for stabilization. In this position the operator may find it more difficult to perceive the transducer-artery angle. During bedside examinations, the operator must always adjust her/his perception of the transducer-artery angle due to changes in her/his position. Additionally, bedside examinations will be technically easier to perform if the operator uses a remote control unit.

The use of stereo headphones is recommended when performing TCDI examinations. Headphones eliminate extraneous noise, providing the operator the optimal environment to detect subtle changes associated with the Doppler signals during the examination.

At the end of the examination, the ultrasound gel should be removed from the patient. Excess gel should be removed from the ultrasound transducer and it should be cleaned using a disinfectant.

Examination Sites

There are four ultrasound pathways ("windows") allowing access to the intracranial arteries. A complete TCDI examination incorporates the following approaches:

1. **Transtemporal**
2. **Transorbital**
3. **Suboccipital**
4. **Submandibular**

The placement of the transducer for the four approaches is illustrated in Figure 4-6. The intracranial arteries evaluated by each approach are listed in Table 4-1. Technical hints used to locate the ultrasound windows are presented first, followed by a more detailed discussion of each ultrasound approach.

Ultrasound Windows

Finding the proper ultrasound window occasionally may be difficult and time consuming. The ultrasound beam needs to penetrate either the temporal bone or a natural cranial ostium, and to intercept the small intracranial arteries in a specific location. Time and patience are essential in identifying optimal TCDI windows so that information will be received by the transducer and good quality Doppler spectral waveforms will be produced.

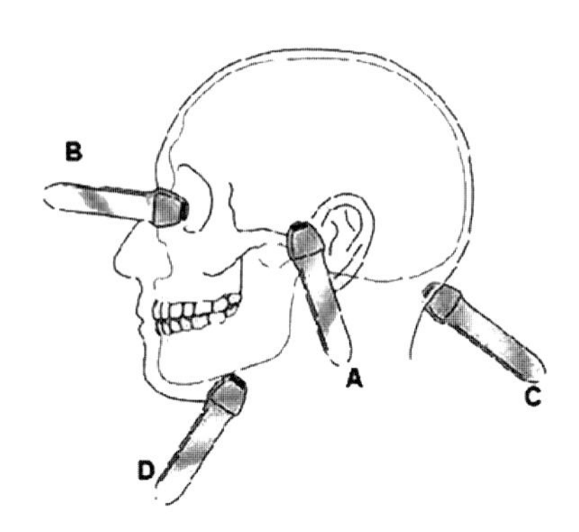

Figure 4-6. Transducer position for the four TCDI windows used during a complete examination. A) Transtemporal, B) Transorbital, C) Suboccipital, and D) Submandibular. [From: Katz ML. Intracranial Cerebrovascular Evaluation. In: Textbook of Diagnostic Ultrasonography. Mosby, St. Louis, 2001]

Table 4-1. The transcranial Doppler windows and the intracranial arteries.

Window	Artery
Transtemporal	Middle Cerebral
	Anterior Cerebral
	Anterior Communicating
	Terminal Internal Carotid
	Posterior Cerebral
	Posterior Communicating
Transorbital	Ophthalmic
	Internal Carotid (siphon)
Suboccipital	Vertebral
	Basilar
Submandibular	Distal Internal Carotid

If a color Doppler signal is located upon initial skin contact, then minimal movement or angling of the transducer maximizes the quality of the ultrasound signal. If a color Doppler signal is not immediately appreciated, and the instrument control settings are correct, then several technical maneuvers can be performed.

Changing the angle of the transducer, thereby redirecting the ultrasound beam, often helps in locating an ultrasound window. The importance of angling the transducer becomes apparent when the variation in size, location, and tortuousity of the intracranial arteries are considered. When angling the transducer to obtain the best quality color Doppler and Doppler signal, part of the face of the transducer is often elevated off the surface of the skin. Additional ultrasound gel may be needed in these cases to maintain good transducer-gel contact.

Simply adjusting the location of the transducer is all that is needed in some patients to find a good ultrasound window. The transducer, however, should be moved slowly over the skin's surface. Moving the transducer 1-2 millimeters frequently finds the window and/or significantly improves the quality of the color Doppler signal. While adjusting the transducer's position, good transducer-gel contact must be maintained.

The depth setting of the sample volume is another important parameter to adjust when locating the ultrasound window. This will vary with each TCDI approach. The depth setting should be adjusted to one that has a high probability of insonating the desired intracranial artery from the approach being used. Since there are differences in the size and shape of patients' heads, and variations of the intracranial arterial anatomy, the sample volume depth setting should be adjusted when searching for an optimal window. Most operators find that the combination of altering the transducer's angle and/or location, and the depth of the sample volume is very rewarding when trying to locate a TCDI window.

As mentioned, good transducer-gel-skin contact is important, and can be obtained with minimal pressure by the transducer. Excessive pressure may create patient discomfort causing anxiety and movement, and may push the ultrasound gel from beneath the transducer causing the Doppler signal to be lost. Proper pressure eliminates interposed air and maintains gel contact between the transducer and skin. When performing TCDI examinations, the patient's hair may also prevent good transducer-gel-skin contact. If a good Doppler signal is not obtained, additional ultrasound gel should be applied to compensate for this minor problem. At the end of the TCDI examination, the ultrasound gel should be removed from the patient, and the ultrasound transducer should be cleaned with a disinfectant.

Technique

The TCD nonimaging (freehand) technique was described in detail in Chapter 3. This chapter addresses specific technical nuances unique to TCDI. The standard transtemporal, transorbital, suboccipital, and submandibular windows are used for transcranial color Doppler imaging. The imaging transducer approved for the transorbital approach will vary with each manufacturer.

Interpretation criteria previously developed with the nonimaging TCD technique are used with TCDI. Color Doppler imaging, however, permits identification of structural landmarks that assist in accurately identifying the intracranial arteries. Anatomic landmarks that are helpful in locating the circle of Willis when using the transtemporal approach are: the petrous ridge of the temporal bone, the sphenoid bone, cerebral falx, supracellar cistern, and the cerebral peduncles. When performing the suboccipital approach, the foramen magnum and the occipital bone are used as anatomic landmarks to locate the vertebrobasilar system. The globe and optic nerve are helpful anatomic landmarks for locating the ophthalmic artery and the carotid siphon when using the transorbital window.

Conventional color orientation for TCDI examinations is set for shades of red indicating blood flow toward the transducer and shades of blue indicating blood flow away from the transducer. By keeping this color assignment constant, intracranial blood flow direction in the arteries can be readily recognized. The appearance of intracranial arterial blood flow is dependent upon many instrument controls that can affect its presentation. Therefore, estimations of arterial size are not accurate from the color Doppler display.

The Doppler evaluation of the intracranial arteries is performed with a large sample volume to obtain a good signal-to-noise ratio. With TCDI, a smaller gate (i.e. 5-10 mm) can be placed on a specific arterial segment that is readily identified from a color flow image. Intracranial arterial velocities acquired with TCDI are acquired assuming a zero degree angle. Several investigators have evaluated the potential use of angle adjusted (corrected) velocities during TCDI.[4-7] Because the walls of the arteries cannot be visualized during TCDI, the operator must angle correct for the color display. Angle adjusted velocities are elevated compared to velocities taken assuming a zero degree angle. Considering that an intracranial artery is tortuous and lies in different ultrasound imaging planes, angle adjustment is only possible for a short segment of the artery.[8] Although the data for angle adjustment appears interesting, it has not been thoroughly evaluated and it is recommended that routine TCDI be performed assuming a zero degree angle.

Additionally, with the use of TCDI, many investigators are reporting results using peak systolic and end diastolic velocities instead of the traditionally accepted mean velocities (time average peak velocities). Each institution will have to decide which velocity value to report, and adjust diagnostic criteria accordingly.

Transtemporal Window

The transtemporal approach is performed with the patient in the supine position and her/his head straight. The transducer is placed on the temporal bone cephalad to the zygomatic arch, and anterior to the ear. A generous amount of acoustic gel is necessary to ensure good transducer-to-skin contact, especially in patients where angling the transducer to optimize the Doppler signal requires the transducer's footprint to be elevated from the skin's surface.

Finding this window can be difficult, and at time frustrating, because ultrasound penetration of the temporal bone is required. Other windows used during the TCDI examination are usually less difficult to find because natural ostia allow easy intracranial penetration of the ultrasound beam. The transtemporal window varies in size and location with each patient, and may vary in an individual from one side to the other. Attenuation of the Doppler signal occurs at the temporal bone interface and its magnitude depends on the thickness of the bone. The ability to penetrate the temporal bone is influenced by the patient's age, sex, and race.[9-13] Hyperostosis of the skull is commonly found in older individuals, females, and in African-Americans. A transtemporal window is not located in up to 30% of the population when performing a TCDI examination.

The transtemporal approach has been described as being divided into three locations over the temporal bone: the anterior, mid, and posterior temporal windows. The posterior transtemporal window is located superior to the zygomatic arch and anterior to the ear, with the transducer aimed in a slightly anterior direction. The anterior transtemporal window is just posterior to the frontal process of the zygoma, and a slight posterior angulation of the transducer is required for accurate insonation. The ultrasound beam is directed medially to properly access the mid transtemporal window, which is located between the anterior and posterior windows.

The mid and posterior transtemporal windows are used more frequently than the anterior window. The mid-transtemporal window is the ideal location because the terminal ICA bifurcation, which is the TCDI reference signal, can be detected by aiming directly medial with the transducer. Each transtemporal window can be used to obtain accurate velocity data if the angle of the transducer is considered in searching for the intracranial arteries. It is important, therefore, to systematically evaluate the entire region so that good quality Doppler signals can be obtained from the best temporal position. It may also be useful during a TCDI examination via the transtemporal window to change the position of the transducer to obtain the best Doppler signal from each of the intracranial arteries.

The transducer's orientation marker/light (this is transducer dependent and varies with the different imaging systems) should be pointing in the anterior direction, with the transducer angled slightly superiorly. This orientation of the transducer produces an imaging plane that is a transverse oblique view that has the advantage of simultaneous visualization of the anterior and posterior intracranial circulation in many patients. The ipsilateral hemisphere is at the top and the contralateral hemisphere at the bottom of the monitor, with anterior being to the left and posterior to the right side (Figure 4-7). With a good transtemporal window and a deep depth setting (14-16 cm), the contralateral skull produces echoes near the bottom of the image.

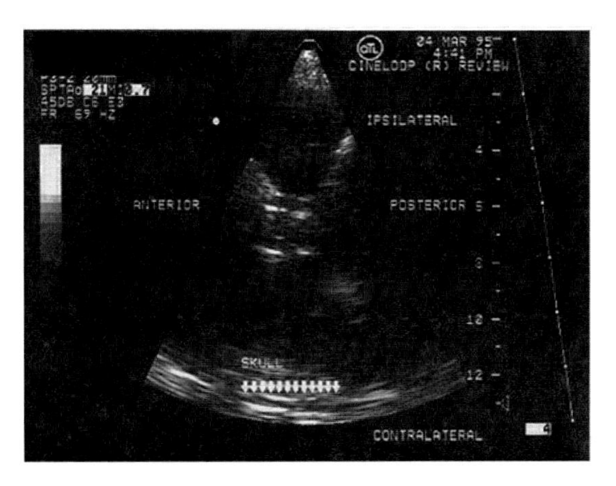

Figure 4-7. Image orientation shown above is from the transtemporal window. Anterior is to the left and posterior to the right side of the image. The ipsilateral hemisphere is at the top of the image. The contralateral skull (arrows) can be visualized near the bottom of the monitor.

The transducer should be angled and moved slowly along the skin surface to find the best transtemporal window. Once located, the image depth setting is adjusted to a depth range of 8-10 cm. Visualization of the contralateral arterial system is possible in many patients, but each hemisphere should be separately studied through ipsilateral windows to obtain the best artery-to-transducer angle. In patients with only a unilateral transtemporal window however, evaluating the contralateral hemisphere is possible and may provide valuable information.

After locating the transtemporal window, the transducer is angled slightly inferior to identify the bony landmarks. These anatomic structures ensure the operator that s/he is at the correct level within the skull to locate the circle of Willis. The reflective echo extending anteriorly is the lesser wing of the sphenoid bone, and the petrous ridge of the temporal bone extends posteriorly (Figure 4-8). The foramen lacerum may be visualized in patients and appears as a small oval echolucent area near the center of the reflective echoes from the bony landmarks. The ipsilateral temporal lobe is at the top of the image. After obtaining visualization of these intracranial landmarks, the gray scale is optimized using the overall gain and times gain compensation (TGC) controls.

The color control is turned on and examination is begun by visualizing the terminal ICA as it courses near the foramen lacerum (Figure 4-9). The mean velocity is normally 39 $\pm$ 9 cm/sec, and the direction of blood flow depends upon the artery's anatomic configuration. In this location, there may be mirror imaging artifact due to the adjacent bone.

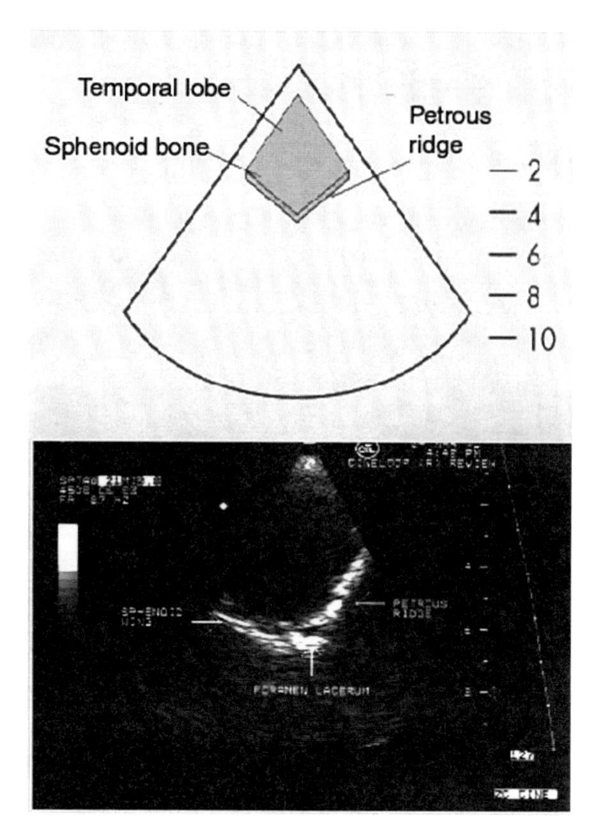

Figure 4-8. A schematic and gray scale image of the bony landmarks visualized from the transtemporal approach. [From: Katz ML. Intracranial Cerebrovascular Evaluation. In: Textbook of Diagnostic Ultrasonography.Mosby, St. Louis, 2001]

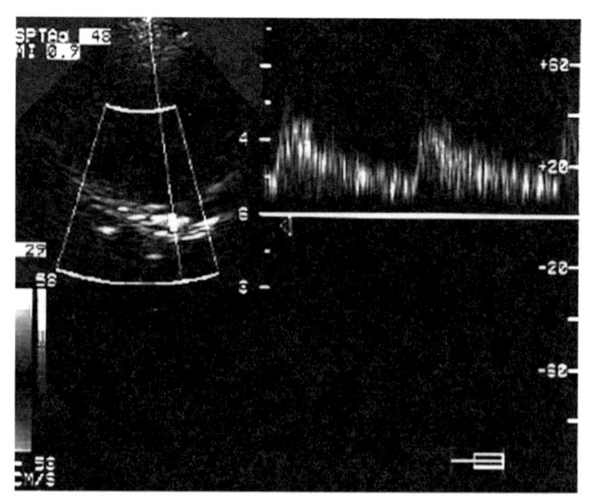

Figure 4-9. The terminal-ICA is visualized from the transtemporal approach.

The transducer is then angled anteriorly and superiorly so that the remainder of the anterior circulation (middle and anterior cerebral arteries) can be examined (Figure 4-10). The sphenoid wing can be used as a bony landmark since the (MCA) courses adjacent to it. The main trunk of the MCA is displayed in red since blood flow is normally toward the transducer. The mean velocity is normally 62 $\pm$ 12 cm/sec. The M2 branches are usually displayed in red but may appear blue as they curve and blood flows away from the transducer.

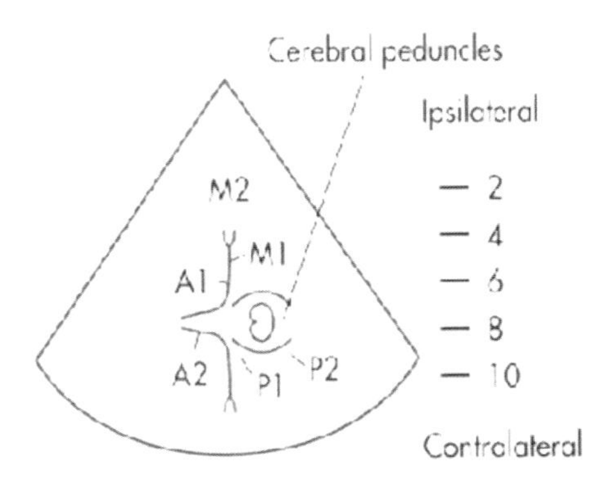

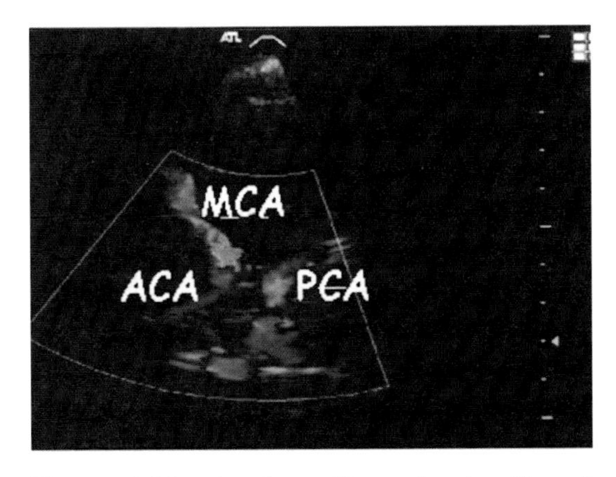

Figure 4-10. A schematic and color Doppler image of the circle of Willis visualized from the transtemporal approach. Note that the contralateral arteries are displayed in the opposite colors. [From: Katz ML. Intracranial Cerebrovascular Evaluation. In: Textbook of Diagnostic Ultrasonography. Mosby, St. Louis, 2001]

The anterior cerebral artery (ACA) is displayed in shades of blue as it courses away from the transducer toward the midline. The transducer may need to be angled slightly anterior and superiorly to visualize the ACA. The mean velocity is normally 50 $\pm$ 11 cm/sec, and the color PRF may need to be decreased to visualize this artery due to its lower velocity. Although not part of the routine TCDI examination, the initial portion of the A2 segment often can be visualized and is displayed in blue extending in an anterior direction at midline into the interhemispheric fissure.

The posterior circulation is visualized by angling the transducer slightly posterior and inferiorly using the cerebral peduncles as an anatomic landmark (Figure 4-11). Normally, the two cerebral peduncles are identical in size and shape, and are of intermediate echogenicity. The posterior cerebral artery (PCA) wraps around the cerebral peduncle (Figure 4-12). The P1 segment of the posterior cerebral artery is displayed in red because blood flow is normally toward the transducer. The color PRF may need to be decreased to visualize the PCAs due to the lower blood flow velocities. The normal mean velocity is 39 $\pm$ 10 cm/sec. The P2 segment of the PCA may be displayed in red (toward the transducer) just distal to the origin of the posterior communicating artery, but will be displayed in blue distally as it wraps around the cerebral peduncle. This is variable due to the vessel tortuousity and orientation to the transducer. Often the ipsilateral and contralateral P1 segments can be visualized at their origin as the basilar artery terminates. The ipsilateral P1 segment is in shades of red and the contralateral P1 segment is displayed in shades of blue.

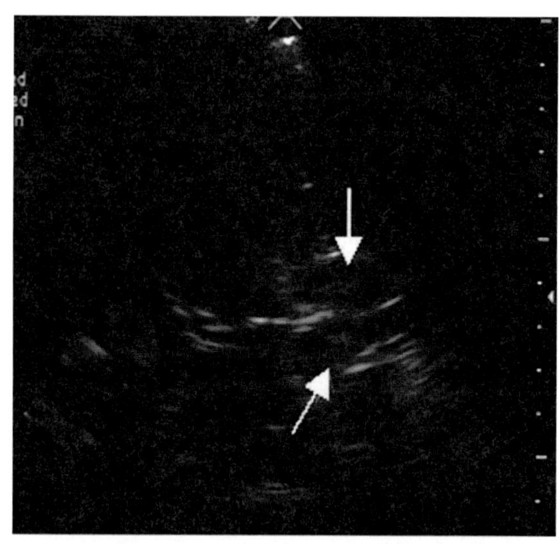

Figure 4-11. The cerebral peduncles (arrows) are visualized from the transtemporal window.

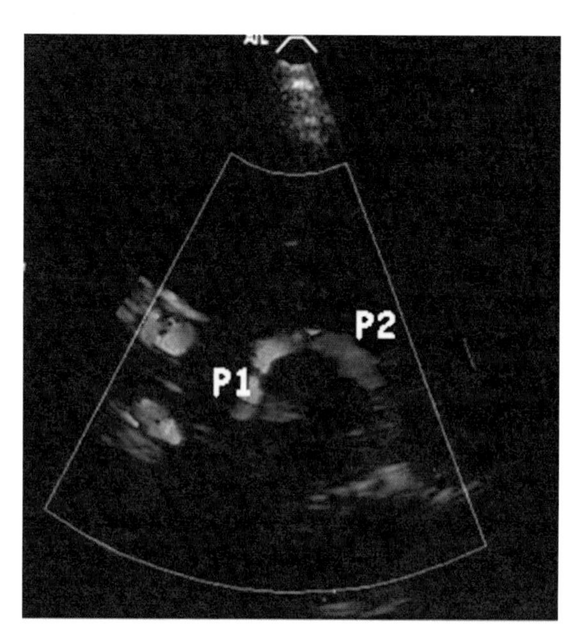

Figure 4-12. The posterior cerebral artery is visualized from the transtemporal approach. The P1 and P2 segments of the PCA are visualized in this TCDI examination.

The anterior communicating artery (ACoA) is not visualized because it is short in length. However, the posterior communicating (PCoA) is longer in length and often is visualized connecting the anterior and posterior circulations in patients (Figure 4-13). The mean peak velocity in the PCoA is 36 ± 15 cm/sec and the direction of blood flow may be toward or away from the transducer. The color PRF may need to be decreased to visualize the PCoA. Additionally, using power Doppler imaging may be helpful in locating the PCoA because this artery often courses parallel to the skin line.

The ability to detect the PCoA with transcranial color Doppler imaging was evaluated by Klotzsch and colleagues.[14] Fifty normal subjects were imaged, and the PCoA was detected unilaterally in 70% (35/50) and bilaterally in 30% (15/50). Blood flow direction was from the PCA to the ICA in 75% (49/65) of the PCoAs identified by transcranial color Doppler imaging. Blood flow direction was from the ICA to the PCA in the remaining 25% (16/65).

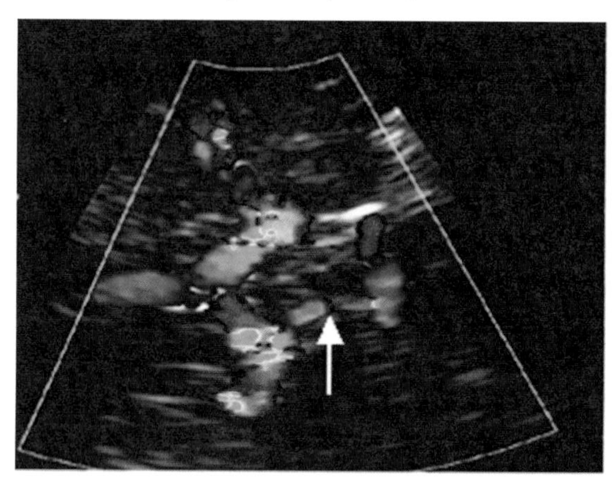

Figure 4-13. The contralateral posterior communicating artery (arrow) is visualized connecting the anterior and posterior circulations via the transtemporal window.

Additionally, Klotzsch and colleagues studied fifteen patients who had undergone unilateral balloon occlusion of the ICA for treatment of intracavernous aneurysms and fifteen patients with unilateral ICA occlusions. TCDI identified bilateral PCoAs in 83% (25/30) and unilateral PCoAs in 17% (5/30). Blood flow direction in the PCoA was from the PCA to the ICA on the ipsilateral side of the ICA occlusion in all thirty patients and in 76% (19/25) of the detectable PCoAs on the contralateral side. The average peak velocity recorded from the PCoA on the ipsilateral side of the ICA occlusion was 64 ± 10 cm/sec compared to 27 ± 14 cm/sec on the contralateral side ($p<0.001$). In 24 of the 30 patients, TCD imaging results were compared to arteriography. TCDI had an overall accuracy of 89.6% in correctly identifying a patent PCoA and determining blood flow direction.

Although the anterior and posterior circulations can be simultaneously visualized in many patients, often the patient's anatomy requires separate evaluation. Minor changes in the transducer's position on the skin or its angle permits individual evaluation of either the anterior or posterior intracranial circulations.

The quality of the intracranial image is dependent upon proper adjustment of many instrument controls. Increasing the color gain to the appropriate level during a TCDI study is probably the most important instrument control adjustment. Adjusting the focal zone in the range of 6-8 cm will improve the image and color resolution. Maintaining a small image sector width and color box width will keep the highest possible frame rates. Checking for the appropriate color PRF, sensitivity, and persistence settings are also very important to obtain good quality color Doppler intracranial images.

The color display is important because it assists in the proper placement of the Doppler sample volume. ***The interpretation of the TCDI examination is made from the Doppler spectral waveform information.*** Therefore, Doppler signals are obtained from various depths along the artery's path. The color Doppler display helps guide the operator, as the Doppler sample volume is "swept" through the , MCA, ACA, and the PCA to obtain the Doppler spectral waveforms. At each depth setting it is important to adjust the position of the sample volume on the color display and angle the transducer to optimize the Doppler signal.

It is important to remember that the transcranial color Doppler images are only in two dimensions. Tortuous intracranial arteries frequently cannot be displayed along their length as a continuous color pathway. In these instances, the gray scale image and color pixel information guides movement of the sample volume through the anatomically correct location, and the operator uses the imaging transducer to obtain the hemodynamic information similar to performing a nonimaging TCD examination.

Suboccipital Window

When evaluating the vertebro-basilar system, the best results are obtained with the patient lying on her/his side with her/his head bowed slightly toward the chest. This position increases the gap between the cranium and the atlas. The orientation marker/light on the transducer should be pointing to the patient's right side and the transducer placed on the posterior aspect of the neck inferiorly to the nuchal crest. The best images from the suboccipital approach are found with the transducer slightly off midline, with the ultrasound beam directed toward the bridge of the patient's nose. When compared to the nonimaging TCD approach for this window, the imaging transducer (wide ultrasound beam) is placed more inferiorly on the neck and angled more superiorly to obtain images of the vertebrobasilar arterial system.

The large circular anaechoic area visualized from this approach is the foramen magnum, and the bright echogenic reflection is from the occipital bone. The depth of these anatomic structures will vary with each patient depending upon the thickness of the suboccipital soft tissue. When these anatomic landmarks have been located, the gray scale image is optimized using image gain and TGC controls. The color control is turned on, and the right vertebral artery will be displayed on the left of the image (monitor) and the left vertebral artery is on the right side (Figure 4-14). The basilar artery is deep (bottom of the image) to the vertebral arteries. The depth range of the image should be set for 10-12 cms. Blood flow in the vertebrobasilar system is normally away from the transducer (Figure 4-15), so the arteries should be displayed in shades of blue.

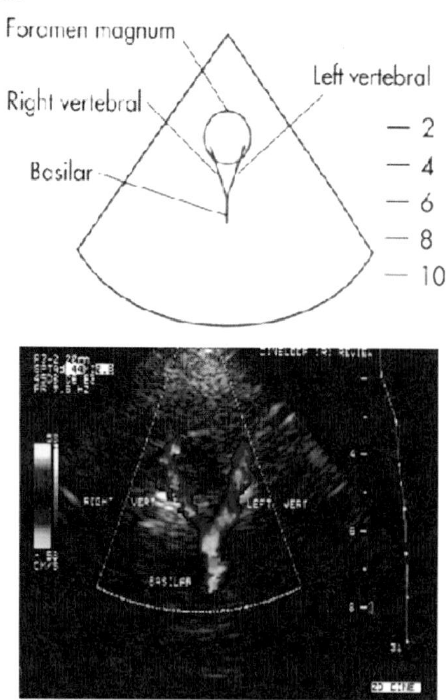

Figure 4-14. A schematic and color Doppler image visualized from the suboccipital approach. The vertebrobasilar system appears as a blue "Y". [From: Katz ML. Intracranial Cerebrovascular Evaluation. In: Textbook of Diagnostic Ultrasonography. Mosby, St. Louis, 2001]

The vertebrobasilar system appears as a blue "Y" on the image. The operator may not always be able to visualize the vertebrobasilar system as a continuous "Y" due to the tortuousity associated with the vertebral and basilar arteries. Even if a "Y"-sign is visualized with color flow imaging, the most distal part of the basilar artery may not be properly displayed from this imaging plane. The basilar artery is often tortuous and visualization of its distal position requires an additional "dig-in" maneuver with the transducer. Relative to the "Y"-sign plane, an operator needs to move the transducer slightly inferiorly but aim more rostrally to visualize the course of the distal basilar artery. An important rule to remember is that the distal basilar artery is usually found at 10 cm depths whereas the "Y"-junction of the vertebral arteries is usually found from 7 - 8.5 cm.

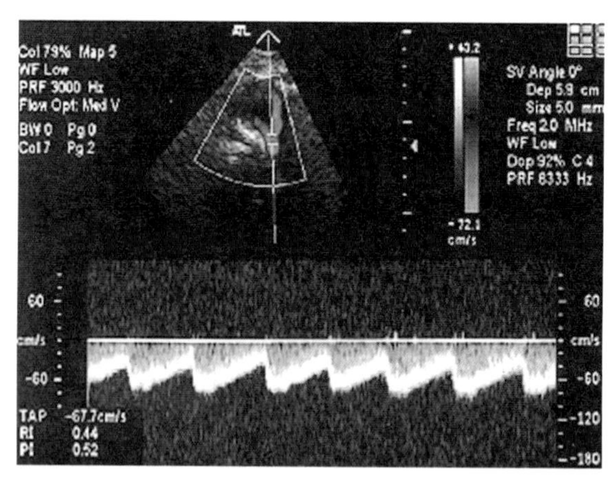

Figure 4-15. The Doppler spectral waveform obtained from the basilar artery. The mean velocity is 68 cm/sec and blood flow is away from the transducer.

The Doppler sample volume is placed in a vertebral artery and the spectral Doppler waveform information is obtained. The sample volume can be moved from side to side or can be swept through each vertebral artery individually. The mean velocity in the vertebral arteries is normally 38 $\pm$ 10 cm/

sec, and the mean velocity is 41 ± 10 cm/sec in the basilar artery. Since the posterior circulation has lower velocities than the anterior circulation, the operator may need to decrease the color PRF to visualize the vertebrobasilar system. Additionally, the operator may need to adjust the transducer's position on the neck or its angle when trying to locate the deeper distal basilar artery. Moving the transducer slightly inferiorly on the neck and angling superiorly often allows better visualization of the distal basilar artery. Following the basilar artery distally (deep), the operator may not visualize color Doppler information. In this case, the operator may use the imaging transducer to obtain the Doppler hemodynamic information similar to performing a nonimaging TCD examination. The sample volume is moved along the expected course of the basilar artery. The terminal portion of the basilar artery as it bifurcates into the PCAs cannot be visualized from this approach.

TCDI allows visualization of the confluence of the vertebral arteries into the basilar artery. The vertebral artery confluence often has been difficult to accurately locate using the nonimaging TCD technique. Several investigators have reported that the average depth of the vertebral artery confluence is approximately 70 ± 7 mm.[15,16] It is important to have properly adjusted color controls when measuring the depth of the vertebral artery confluence. If the color gain is too high, the color will extend into the surrounding brain tissue and the confluence may appear more superficial. Additionally, branches of the vertebral arteries, especially the posterior inferior cerebellar artery (PICA), often can be visualized and are usually displayed in red as they curve and carry blood toward the transducer.

Transorbital Window

The transorbital evaluation provides information about the ophthalmic artery and the carotid siphon.[17-20] The United States Food and Drug Administration (FDA) has approved certain imaging transducers on various manufacturers' equipment for the evaluation of the orbit. It is important for each operator to contact the appropriate ultrasound manufacturing company and determine which transducer is approved for orbital imaging for their imaging system.

It is important when imaging the orbit to decrease the power setting significantly prior to evaluating the orbit. Using a low power output, successful color Doppler imaging of the orbit has been reported. Additionally, the examination time should be minimized. Although there are not any known observed bioeffects from the ultrasound evaluation of the eye, the power settings of color Doppler imaging systems raise concern for ocular damage. The current FDA maximum acoustic output allowable levels (derated) for ophthalmic imaging are a spatial peak temporal average (SPTA) intensity of 17 mW/cm^2 and a mechanical index (MI) of 0.28. The guiding principle for the use of diagnostic ultrasound is the ALARA ("as low as reasonably achievable") principle.

The examination is performed with the patient in the supine position and the transducer gently placed on the closed eyelid. Removal of contact lenses is only necessary for patient comfort. A liberal amount of acoustic gel is important and firm pressure on the eyelid is not necessary or recommended. Careful attention to instrument controls is important to minimize artifacts caused by involuntary eye movement. Sometimes it is helpful to instruct the patient to focus their eyes to the opposite side from that being examined.

The orientation marker on the imaging transducer should be pointed medially, toward the nose, when performing the right or left examination. Examination of either eye produces an image with medial (nasal) on the left side and temporal on the right side of the monitor. A variation of this technique is to have the transducer's orientation marker directed to the patient's right side when evaluating either eye. This transducer orientation will produce an image with medial (nasal) on the monitor's left when examining the left eye and medial on the monitor's right side when evaluating the right eye (Figure 4-16). The globe is at the top of the image (monitor).

The carotid siphon is located at a depth of 60-80 mm and the mean velocity is 47 $\pm$ 14 cm/sec. Direction of blood flow depends on which segment (parasellar, genu, supraclinoid) of the carotid siphon is insonated. Blood flow is bi-directional at the genu, toward the transducer in the parasellar portion, and away from the transducer in the supraclinoid segment.

To evaluate the ophthalmic artery (OA), the depth setting of the Doppler sample volume should be in the range of 40-60mm. A better image of this superficial segment may be obtained using a higher frequency (7.5-10 MHz) linear array transducer. The ultrasound beam should be directed slightly medially along the anterior-posterior plane. The OA is generally identified adjacent to the optic nerve. The color PRF needs to be decreased to visualize the ophthalmic artery and blood flow is normally toward the transducer with a mean velocity of 21 $\pm$ 5 cm/sec. The Doppler signal has a high pulsatility because the OA supplies blood to the globe and its structures.

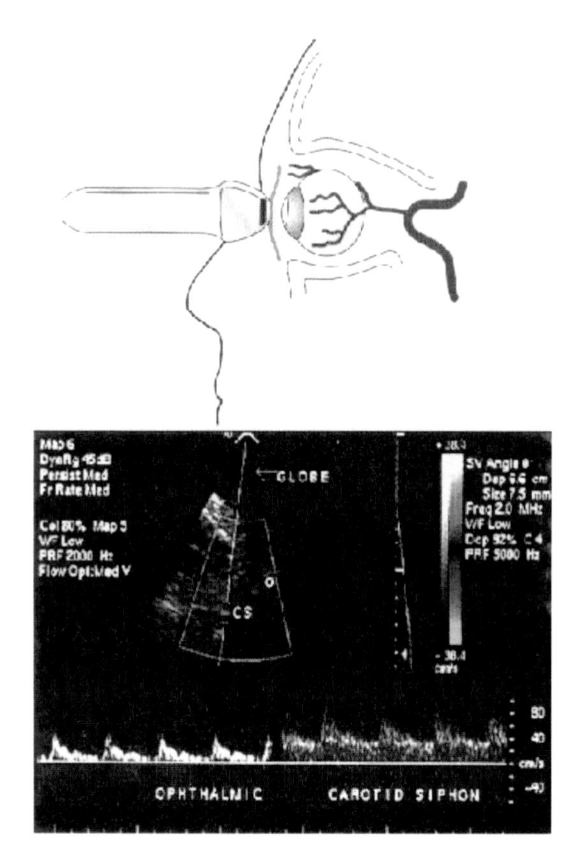

Figure 4-16. A schematic and color Doppler image visualized from the transorbital approach. Note the high resistance Doppler signal from the ophthalmic artery compared to the low resistance Doppler signal from the siphon. [From: Katz ML. Intracranial Cerebrovascular Evaluation. In: Textbook of Diagnostic Ultrasonography. Mosby, St. Louis, 2001]

Submandibular Window

The submandibular approach is a continuation of the duplex imaging evaluation of the extracranial distal. The transducer is placed at the angle of the mandible and angled slightly medially and cephalad toward the carotid canal. The transducer's orientation marker/light is pointed in a superior direction. Distal ICA blood flow is away from the transducer and is displayed in shades of blue. Careful Doppler evaluation will distinguish the ICA's low resistance signal from the higher resistance signal from the ECA. Venous blood flow is less pulsatile and is directed toward the transducer (shades of red) at this location. The transducer's angle should be adjusted to follow the retromandibular portion of the ICA. The mean velocity in this segment of the ICA is normally 37 $\pm$ 9 cm/sec. At the end of the TCDI examination, the ultrasound gel should be removed from the patient. Excess gel should be removed from the ultrasound transducer and it should be cleaned using a disinfectant.

Advantages/Limitations of Transcranial Color Doppler Imaging

TCDI has a number of advantages and limitations when compared to the nonimaging TCD technique (Table 4-2). Reducing the limitations and maximizing the advantages will ensure the most complete evaluation.

A limitation of the TCDI technique includes the operator having a sound understanding of complex color Doppler imaging principles. To obtain a good quality study, this technique involves the proper use of more instrument controls than the nonimaging TCD technique. Imaging systems are larger and, therefore, less portable, causing it to be more cumbersome to move the equipment and perform bedside evaluations in small intensive care rooms or when used in the operating room or radiology suites. Although the distal basilar artery is often difficult to evaluate with the nonimaging TCD technique, imaging of this portion of the artery is rarely possible with color Doppler imaging because of the larger beam width. However, the basilar artery can usually be followed distally by increasing the sample volume depth and continuing the study like a nonimaging examination by using the Doppler signal as a guide. The larger beamwidth may also hamper the penetration of the temporal bone when the transtemporal ultrasound window is small.[21]

Table 4-2. Limitations of the TCDI examination

- Operator experience
- Improper instrument control settings
- Patient movement
- Absent or poor temporal window
- Anatomic variations
- Arterial misidentification
- Distal branch disease
- Distal basilar artery
- Misinterpretation of collateral channels or vasospasm as a stenosis
- Displacement of arteries by an intracranial mass

There are several advantages of using TCDI compared to the nonimaging technique. Imaging allows the bony and soft tissue landmarks to be used as anatomic guides to identify the intracranial arteries quickly and with more accuracy. Additionally, tissue harmonic imaging has been shown to improve the identification of parenchymal structures.[22] This instills confidence in the operator and leads to improved reliability. Using the anatomic landmarks also allows the accurate evaluation of the intracranial arteries if nontraditional window (i.e. posterior to the ear, frontal) are used when the squamous portion of the temporal bone is too thick.[23] With good ultrasound windows, the examination time is reduced since the operator is able to move the sample volume along the path of the artery to obtain the hemodynamic information (Doppler spectral waveforms). Those who are inexperienced with the TCD technique also find that the learning curve is shorter with the TCDI technique.

Additionally, TCDI allows: the identification of the individual large M2 branches (Figure 4-17); the accurate identification of contralateral arteries if a transtemporal window can be located on only one side; collateral pathways are readily identified; tortuous vessels can be followed and evaluated accurately; and the vertebral confluence can be identified in many patients. Imaging provides a method to document the location from which the Doppler spectral waveform is derived, which becomes important with repeat examinations, in departments where there are multiple operators and/or interpreters, and for quality improvement.

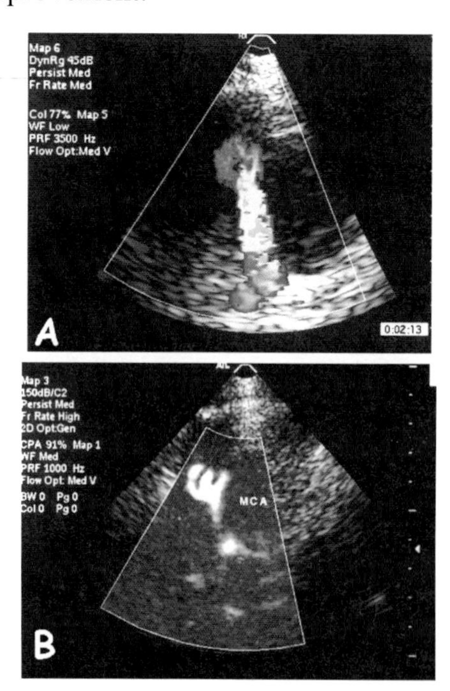

Figure 4-17. The M2 branches of the are displayed in A) color Doppler, and B) with power Doppler imaging.

The introduction of TCDI has expanded the applications of TCD. Weismann and Seidel evaluated two doses (0.5 and 1.5 mL) of Optison (a perfluorpropane-based ultrasound contrast agent) in 13 healthy volunteers.[66] In this study, the investigators were able to calculate color-coded perfusion maps from the ultrasound gray scale imaging data to analyze brain tissue perfusion during bedside examinations. In another study, Seidel and colleagues monitored 23 consecutive patients with repeated TCDI and intracerebral hematomas confirmed with computed tomography (CT).[24] In three patients (13%), there was absence of a transtemporal window. Localization of the hematomas was possible in 18 patients (78%). A small intracortical hemorrhage (1.2 x 0.8 cm^2) was missed in one patient and, in another patient; an extensive hemorrhage into the basal ganglia was misdiagnosed as a lobar hematoma. Additionally, the investigators monitored the change in the sonographic characteristics of the hematomas. Initially, they found the hematoma to appear more homogenously echogenic than the surrounding brain tissue, with a gradual decrease in echogenicity in the center of the hematoma occurring over time. In the subacute state, this appears as a lesion with a hypoechogenic center surrounded by a hyperechogenic margin. The echogenicity decreases over a period of weeks, the margin becomes blurred, and complete resolution appears to occur after a minimum of two to five weeks.

Becker and colleagues investigated using TCDI to differentiate between ischemic and hemorrhagic stroke.[25] Twenty-eight patients with parenchymal hemorrhages, and 20 patients with ischemic stroke, had complete neurologic evaluations including TCDI and CT scan. In six patients, the transtemporal window was absent. The CT diagnosis of parenchymal hemorrhage was confirmed by TCDI in 24 of 28 patients (absence of window in 3 patients). The authors found recent hemorrhage to be echogenic compared to the surrounding brain parenchyma. TCDI was diagnostic in 17 of 20 patients with ischemic stroke (absence of temporal windows in 3 patients). In ischemic infarction, the brain tissue displays no change in echogenicity or echotexture. The diagnosis of ischemic stroke is based on the demonstration of vascular pathology.

Mauer and colleagues also investigated using TCDI to differentiate between intracerebral hemorrhage and ischemic stroke.[26] One hundred and fifty-one patients were enrolled in a prospective study. Each patient had a neurological examination, a CT scan, and a TCDI examination. CT scanning revealed 60 patients with intracerebral hemorrhage, 67 patients with an ischemic stroke, and in 24 patients the CT findings were inconclusive. TCDI was not possible in 18 patients because of the lack of a transtemporal window. Of the remaining 133 patients, TCDI was in agreement with the CT scan in 126 patients. TCDI missed 3 atypical bleedings (2 with an upper parietal location), and in 4 patients without bleeding, an intracerebral hemorrhage was suspected because of increased echogenicity due to microangiopathy. The authors concluded that using transcranial color Doppler imaging is an alternative when CT is not readily available or if the patient cannot be moved.

Similar to nonimaging TCD techniques, color Doppler imaging has been described in the identification of arteriovenous malformations.[27,28] The major afferent feeding vessels and the AVM's venous drainage can be identified with TCDI. The advantage of transcranial color Doppler imaging is that it allows the accurate identification of the different feeding arteries. Repeated measurement with angle adjustment during stepwise embolization is possible. This allows for a precise quantification of the hemodynamic changes that occur during the treatment process. This technique may be helpful in the planning of the different stages of embolization in these patients.

TCDI has been reported to have a sensitivity ranging from 0 to 85% for the identification of cerebral aneurysms.[29-34] Large, non-thrombosed aneurysms were identified, but small aneurysms (less than 5 mm) and thrombosed aneurysms were missed by TCDI. Wardlaw and colleagues described four ultrasound features that assist in the identification of intracranial aneurysms: 1) rounded color areas projecting from an artery that appear noncontinuous at both ends with an artery, 2) color flow appearing in an unexpected area, 3) a color area that is wider than the adjacent arteries, and 4) an area with greater expansion and contraction during the cardiac cycle compared to the adjacent artery.[31] Although TCDI may not be the best method to detect cerebral aneurysms, TCDI operators should be aware of their occurrence and the associated hemodynamic characteristics for potential identification during a TCDI examination.

In addition, TCDI is being used in the identification of intracranial arterial stenosis[35], acute stroke[36-38,67], thrombolytic therapy[39,40], and to screen children with sickle cell disease.[41-42]

TCDI with contrast enhancement has improved the evaluation of the circle of Willis, and the distal basilar artery in patients with inadequate windows.[43-53,68,69] Using contrast enhanced color Doppler imaging has increased the detection of clinically relevant intracranial arterial disease that may influence the further work-up and/ or management of patients. Additionally, detected Doppler spectral waveforms have demonstrated an increase in velocity after the administration of contrast material.[54] This velocity increase may be real or artificial due to better visualization of the Doppler signal. Intracranial arterial velocity criteria may need to be developed for use when performing TCDI with contrast agents.

Intracranial veins

Investigators are exploring the capability of evaluating the intracranial veins by TCDI.[55-62] The venous TCDI evaluation of normal volunteers and in patients with venous sinus thrombosis have been reported.

Several instrument adjustments are important when using TCD equipment to evaluate intracranial venous blood flow. Ultrasound insonation of normal intracranial veins produce low amplitude, pulsatile Doppler signals. Therefore, the pulse repetition frequency and the wall filter settings should be significantly reduced to insure acquisition of good quality intracranial venous Doppler signals.

The basal vein of Rosenthal (BVR) is a prominent basal vein that is located near the P2 segment of the posterior cerebral artery. The BVR produces a low frequency Doppler signal. Blood flow direction is away from the transducer, from the transtemporal approach. The mean depth range for the BVR is 55 to 75 mm and the mean velocity is 10 $\pm$ 2 cm/sec.

The deep middle cerebral vein (dMCV) parallels the middle cerebral artery. Blood flow is away from the transducer from the transtemporal approach. The dMCV is located in the depth range of 45-60 mm and the mean velocity is 11 $\pm$ 3 cm/sec.

The straight sinus is evaluated from the suboccipital approach. The TCDI transducer is directed toward the brain midline and the sample volume depth setting range is from 50 to 70 mm. Blood flow direction is normally toward the transducer and the mean velocity is approximately 20 cm/sec.

The TCDI examination of the intracranial venous system is a new area that is currently being evaluated. Further investigation is necessary prior to establishing the clinical utility of TCDI in the evaluation of the intracranial venous systems. The extension of using TCDI to evaluate the intracranial venous system may allow a new perspective on cerebrovenous disorders.

Summary

TCDI offers new and important advantages to the TCD technique. Using the anatomic landmarks and proper instrument controls, a more accurate and reproducible evaluation of the complex intracranial arterial hemodynamics can be performed (Table 4-3).

The most comprehensive transcranial Doppler evaluation will be performed using the imaging transducer in conjunction with the nonimaging transducer. Color power imaging offers the technical advantage in imaging small caliber intracranial arteries, slower moving blood flow, and in imaging the intracranial arteries that course at unfavorable angles to the ultrasound beam.[63-64]

Future technology may offer improved visualization of the intracranial circulation by using 3-D ultrasound imaging,[65] and color Doppler imaging with contrast enhancement.[43-53]

Table 4-3. Summary: Transcranial color Doppler imaging

- Take a patient history (focus on history, risk factors, and symptoms)
- Be aware of the status of the extracranial vessels
- Be familiar with intracranial arterial anatomy
- Understand how each color control affects the image and how the controls affect each other
- Use the color/power Doppler display as a guide to obtain the Doppler spectral waveform information
- Use a large Doppler sample volume (10-15mm) and assume a zero degree angle
- Be aware of the Doppler spectral waveform configuration
- Compare the Doppler spectral waveforms from the anterior and posterior circulations, and from left and right sides
- Establish institutional diagnostic criteria for the various clinical applications

References

1. Kremkau FW. Doppler Ultrasound: Principles and Instruments. 6th ed. Philadelphia: WB Saunders, 2002.
2. Aaslid R. Transcranial Doppler Examination Techniques. Chapter 4. In: Aaslid R (Ed), Transcranial Doppler Sonography, New York, Springer-Verlag, 1986:39-59.
3. Sound Ergonomics LLC. Consultants for Sonographer Health. Accessed on December 5, 2001. http://soundergonomics.com
4. Tsuchiya T, Yasaka M, Yamaguchi T, et al. Imaging of the basal cerebral arteries and measurement of blood velocity in adults by using transcranial real-time color flow Doppler sonography. AJNR 22: 497-502, 1991.
5. Schoning M, Buchholz R, Walter J. Comparative study of transcranial color duplex sonography and transcranial Doppler sonography in adults. J Neurosurg 78:776-784, 1993.
6. Eicke BM, Tegeler CH, Dalley G, Myers LG. Angle correction in transcranial Doppler sonography. J Neuroimag 4:29-33, 1994.
7. Krejza J, Mariak Z, Babikian VL. Importance of angle correction in the measurement of blood flow velocity with transcranial Doppler sonography. Am J Neuroradiol. 22:1743-1747, 2001.
8. Giller GA. Is angle correction correct? J Neuroimag 4:51-52, 1994.
9. Grolimund P. Transmission of ultrasound through the temporal bone. Chapter 2. In: Aaslid R (Ed), Transcranial Doppler Sonography, pp10-21, New York: Springer-Verlag, 1986.
10. Eden A. Letter to the Editor. Effect of emitted power on waveform intensity in transcranial Doppler. Stroke 22:533, 1991.
11. Halsey JH. Letter to the Editor. Stroke 22:533-534, 1991.

12. Gomez CR, Gomez SM, Hall IS. The elusive transtemporal window: a technical and demographic study. J Cardiovasc Technol 8:1710172, 1989.

13. Marinoni M, Ginanneschi A, Forleo P, Amaducci L. Technical limits in transcranial Doppler recording: Inadequate acoustic windows. Ultrasound Med Biol 23:1275-1277, 1997.

14. Klotzch C, Popescu O, Berlit P. Assessment of the posterior communicating artery by transcranial color-coded duplex sonography. Stroke 27:486-489, 1996.

15. Schoning M, Walter J. Evaluation of the vertebrobasilar-posterior system by transcranial color duplex sonography in adults. Stroke 23:1280-1286, 1992.

16. Kaps M, Seidel G, Bauer T, Behrmann B. Imaging of the intracranial vertebrobasilar system using color-coded ultrasound. Stroke 23:1577-1582, 1992.

17. Lieb WE, Cohen SM, Merton DA, et al. Color Doppler imaging of the eye and orbit. Technique and normal vascular anatomy. Arch Ophthalmol 109:527-531, 1991.

18. Lieb WE, Flaharty PM, Sergott RC, et al. Color Doppler imaging provides accurate assessment of orbital blood flow in occlusive carotid artery disease. Ophthalmology 98:548-552, 1991.

19. Giovagnorio F, Quaranta L, Bucci MG. Color Doppler assessment of normal ocular blood flow. J Ultrasound Med 12:473-477, 1993.

20. Hu H-H, Sheng W-Y, Yen M-Y, et al. Color Doppler imaging of orbital arteries for detection of carotid occlusive disease. Stroke 24:1196-1203, 1993.

21. Fujioka KA, Gates DT, Spenser MP. A comparison of transcranial color Doppler imaging and standard static pulsed wave Doppler in the assessment of intracranial hemodynamics. J Vasc Technol 18:29-35, 1994.

22. Puls I, Berg D, Maurer M, et al. Transcranial sonography of the brain parenchyma: comparison of B-mode imaging and tissue harmonic imaging. Ultrasound in Med & Biol. 26:189-194, 2000.

23. Stolz E, Kaps M, Kern A, Dorndorf W. Frontal bone windows for transcranial color-coded duplex sonography. Stroke 30:814-820, 1999.

24. Seidel G, Kaps M, Dorndor W. Transcranial color-coded duplex sonography of intracerebral hematomas in adults. Stroke 24:1519-1527, 1993.

25. Becker G, Winkler J, Hofmann E, Bogdahn U. Differentiation between ischemic and hemorrhagic stroke by transcranial color-coded real-time sonography. J Neuroimag 3: 41-47, 1993.

26. Mauer M, Shambal S, Berg D, et al. Differentiation between intracerebral hemorrhage and ischemic stroke by transcranial color-coded duplex-sonography. Stroke 29:2563-2567, 1998.

27. Becker GM, Winkler J, Hoffmann E, Bogdahn U. Imaging of cerebral arterio-venous malformations by transcranial colour-coded real-time sonography. Neuroradiology 32:280-288, 1990.

28. Klotzsch C, Henkes H, Nahser HC, et al. Transcranial color-coded duplex sonography in cerebral arteriovenous malformations. Stroke 26:2298-2301, 1995.

29. Baumgartner RW, Mattle HP, et al. Transcranial color-coded duplex sonography in cerebral aneurysms. Stroke 25:2429-2434, 1994.

30. Martin PJ, Gaunt ME, Naylor AR, et al. Intracranial aneurysms and arteriovenous malformations: transcranial colour-coded sonography as a diagnostic aid. Ultrasound Med Biol 20:689-698, 1994.

31. Wardlaw JM, Cannon JC. Color transcranial "power" Doppler ultrasound of intracranial aneurysms. J Neurosurg 84:459-461, 1996.

32. White PM, Wardlaw JM, Teasdale E, et al. Power transcranial Doppler ultrasound in the detection of intracranial aneurysms. Stroke 32:1291-1297, 2001.

33. Becker G, Greiner K, Kuane B, et al. Diagnosis and monitoring of subarachnoid hemorrhage by transcranial color-coded real-time sonography. Neurosurgery 28:814-820, 1991.

34. Becker GM, Greiner K, Kaune B, et al. Diagnosis and monitoring of subarachnoid hemorrhage by transcranial color-coded real-time sonography. Neurosurgery 28:814-820, 1991.

35. Baumgartner RW, Mattle HP, Schroth G. Assessment of =50% and <50% intracranial stenoses by transcranial color-coded duplex sonography. Stroke 30:87-92, 1999.

36. Kenton AR, Martin PJ, Abbott RJ, Moody AR. Comparison of transcranial color-coded sonography and magnetic resonance angiography in acute stroke. Stroke 28:1601-1606, 1997.

37. Goertler M, Kross R, Baeumer M, et al. Diagnostic impact and prognostic relevance of early contrast-enhanced transcranial color-coded duplex sonography in acute stroke. Stroke 29:955-962, 1998.

38. Nabavi DG, Droste DW, Kemeny V, et al. Potential and limitations of echocontrast-enhancedultrasonography in acute stroke patients. A pilot study. Stroke 29:949-954, 1998.

39. Kaps M, Link A. Transcranial sonographic monitoring during thrombolytic therapy. Am J Neuroradiol 19:758-760, 1998.

40. Devuyst G, Afsar N. Is transcranial colour duplex flow imaging of use in selection of patients with acute stroke for thrombolysis? J Neurol Neurosurg Psychiatry 68:794, 2000.

41. Seibert JJ, Glasier CM, Kirby RS, et al. Transcranial Doppler, MRA, and MRI as a screening examination for cerebrovascular disease in patients with sickle cell anemia: an 8-year study. Pediatr Radiol 28:138-142, 1998.

42. Jones AM, Seibert JJ, Nichols FT et al. Comparison of transcranial color Doppler imaging (TCDI) and transcranial Doppler (TCD) in children with sickle-cell anemia. Pediatr Radiol 31:461-469, 2001.

43. Ries F, Kaal K, Schultheiss R, et al. Air microbubbles as a contrast medium in transcranial Doppler sonography. J Neuroimag 1:173-178, 1991.

44. Ries F, Honisch C, Lambertz M, Schlief R. A transpulmonary contrast medium enhances the transcranial Doppler signal in humans. Stroke 24: 1903-1909, 1993.

45. Bogdahn U, Becker G, Schlief R, et al. Contrast-enhanced transcranial color-coded real-time sonography. Stroke 24: 676-684, 1993.

46. Otis S, Rush M, Boyajian R. Contrast-enhanced transcranial imaging. Results of an American phase-two study. Stroke 26:203-209, 1995.

47. Kaps M, Schaffer P, Beller K-D, Seidel G. Transcranial Doppler echo contrast studies using different colour processing modes. Acta Neurol Scand 95:358-362, 1997.

48. Ries F. Clinical experience with echo-enhanced transcranial Doppler and duplex imaging. J of Neuroimaging 7 (suppl 1):S15-S21, 1997.

49. Burns PN. Overview of echo-enhanced vascular ultrasound imaging for clinical diagonsis in neurosonology. J of Neuroimaging 7 (suppl 1):S2-S14, 1997.

50. Kaps M, Schaffer P, Beller K-D, et al. Characteristics of transcranial Doppler signal enhancement using a phosolipid-containing echocontrast agent. Stroke 28:1006-1008, 1997.

51. Iglseder B, Huemer M, Staffen W, Ladurner G. Imaging the basilar artery by contrast-enhanced color-coded ultrasound. J Neuroimaging 10:195-199, 2000.

52. Gahn G, Gerber J, Hallmeyer S, et al. Contrast-enhanced transcranial color-coded duplex sonography in stroke patients with limited bone windows. Am J Neuroradiol 21:509-514, 2000.

53. Uggowitzer MM, Kugler C, Riccabona M, et al. Cerebral arteriovenous malformations: diagnostic value of echo-enhanced transcranial Doppler sonography compared with angiography. Am J Neuroradiol 20:101-106, 1999.

54. Khan HG, Gailloud P, Bude RO, et al. The effect of contrast material on transcranial Doppler evaluation of normal peak systolic velocity. Am J Neuroradiol 21:386-390, 2000.

55. Becker G, Bogdahn U, Gehlberg C, et al. Transcranial color-coded real-time sonography of intracranial veins. Normal values of blood flow velocities and findings in superior sagittal sinus thrombosis. J Neuroimag 5: 87-94, 1995.

56. Valdueza JM, Schultz M, Harms L, Einhaupl KM. Venous transcranial Doppler ultrasound monitoring in acute dural sinus thrombosis. Report of two cases. Stroke 26:1196-1199, 1995.

57. Valdueza JM, Schmierer K, Mehraein S, Einhaupl KM. Assessment of normal flow velocity in basal cerebral veins. A transcranial Doppler ultrasound study. Stroke 27: 1221-1225, 1996.

58. Baumgartner RW, Nirkko AC, Muri RM, Gonner F. Transoccipital power-based color-coded duplex sonography of cerebral sinuses and veins. Stroke 28:1319-1323, 1997.

59. Valdueza JM, Harms L, Doepp F, et al. Venous microembolic signals detected in patients with cerebral sinus thrombosis. Stroke 28:1607-1609, 1997.

60. Stolz E, Kaps M, Dorndorf W. Assessment of intracranial venous hemodynamics in normal individuals and patients with cerebral venous thrombosis. Stroke 30:70-75, 1999.

61. Stolz E, Babacan SS, Bodeker RH, et al. Interobserver and intraobserver reliability of venous transcranial color-coded flow velocity measurements. J Neuroimaging 11:385-92, 2001.

62. Ries S, Steinke W, Neff KW, Hennerici M. Echocontrast-enhanced transcranial color-coded sonography for the diagnosis of transverse sinus venous thrombosis. Stroke 28:696-700, 1997.

63. Baumgartner RW, Schmid C, Baumgartner I. Comparative study of power-based versus mean frequency-based transcranial color-coded duplex sonography in normal adults. Stroke 27:101-104, 1996.

64. Kenton AR, Martin PJ, Evans DH. Power Doppler: An advance over colour Doppler for transcranial imaging? Ultrasound in Med & Biol 22:313-317, 1996.

65. Lyden PD, Nelson TR. Visualization of the cerebral circulation using three-dimensional transcranial power Doppler ultrasound imaging. J of Neuroimaging 7:35-39, 1997.

66. Weismann M, Seidel G. Ultrasound perfusion imaging of the human brain. Stroke 31:2421-2425, 2000.

67. Gerriets T, Goertler M, Stolz E, et al. Feasibility and validity of transcranial duplex sonography in patients with acute stroke. J Neurol Neurosurg Psychiatry 73:17-20, 2002.

68. Stolz E, Nuckel M, Mendez I, et al. Vertebrobasilar transcranial color-coded duplex ultrasonography: improvement with echo enhancement. AJNR 23:1051-1054, 2002.

69. Zunker P, Wilms H, Brossman J, et al. Echo contrast-enhanced transcranial ultrasound: frequency of use, diagnostic benefit, and validity of results compared with MRA. Stroke 33:2600-2603, 2002..

Chapter 5
Normal Values And Physiological Variables

Standard interpretation criteria for transcranial Doppler (TCD) examinations have been reported in the literature. During the evolution of the TCD examination, however, it became obvious that underlying physiologic variables affect the intracranial velocities. Therefore, it is important to be aware of the factors that may affect intracranial hemodynamics and interpret each case individually.

This chapter describes: 1) TCD criteria to identify intracranial arteries, 2) normal velocity ranges, and 3) physiologic factors that influence the TCD spectral waveforms.

Artery Identification

Proper identification of the intracranial vasculature is, of course, the first step in evaluating the TCD examination. Each TCD window provides access to specific arteries, and the identification of the intracranial arteries is based upon the following six criteria:

1. Depth of the sample volume
2. Angle (spatial orientation) of the transducer
3. Direction of blood flow relative to the transducer
4. Spatial relationship of one Doppler signal to another
5. Traceability of an artery
6. Signal response to compression/ vibration maneuvers*

** CCA compression is <u>not</u> routinely required for arterial identification if the other five criteria are applied.*

Sample Volume Depth

The depth of the sample volume is a key criterion to identify intracranial arteries. It is measured in millimeters (mm), and is the distance from the face of the TCD transducer to the middle of the Doppler sample volume. The sample volume length is larger in TCD instruments, usually in the range of 10-15 mm, to achieve a better signal-to-noise ratio. Think about depth and sample volume as mean and standard deviations. For example, if you set the depth of insonation at 50 mm with a sample volume size of 10 mm, you can detect flow signals anywhere from 45 to 55 mm (depth +/- half of the sample volume). Note that 90% of signals usually originate within a 3 mm core of the sample volume, i.e. closely around the set depth. The depths at which the intracranial arteries can be located from each TCD window are listed in Table #5-1. The depths of the arteries may vary with each individual, but in most adults, the sought after artery will usually fall within these ranges. Midline is usually found in the range of 70-80 mm in most adults.

Transducer Angle

The angle of the transducer, or its spatial orientation relative to skull structures, is also important since different intracranial arteries can be insonated at the same depth from a TCD ultrasound window. The angle of the transducer is key in the correct identification of the arteries during a TCD examination. The operator must be able to judge the transducer's relation to the patient's head, and to perceive the normal location of the intracranial arteries. This can be a difficult skill to learn, and can be challenging due to the anatomic variability of the intracranial arteries. The operator's position at the head of

the patient will enable the best perception of the transducer-artery angle. This allows the operator to have access to both sides of the patient's head, and also permits orientation of the TCD transducer to the body's axes and planes.

Table 5-1. Intracranial arterial identification criteria

Window	Artery	Depth (mm)	Direction*
Transtemporal	MCA	30-67	Toward
	ACA	60-80	Away
	t-ICA	55-67	Toward
	PCA	55-75	Toward
Transorbital	Ophthal	40-60	Toward
	ICA siphon	60-80	Bi,Away, towards
Suboccipital	Vertebral	40-85	Away
	Basilar	>80	Away
Submandibular	ICA	35-70	Away

*** Direction is relative to the TCD transducer. MCA: middle cerebral artery, ACA: anterior cerebral artery, t-ICA: terminal internal carotid artery, PCA: posterior cerebral artery, ICA: internal cerebral artery, Ophth: Ophthalmic artery, Vert: vertebral artery, Bi: bi-directional.**

Blood Flow Direction

The normal direction of blood flow in the intracranial arteries relative to the transducer are listed in Table 5-1. From the different TCD approaches, Doppler spectral waveforms may demonstrate blood flow direction away from, toward, or in both directions (bi-directional). If the direction of blood flow is reversed from the established norm, it can be assumed that the artery is functioning as a collateral channel or that there may be an anatomic variant.

Spatial Relationship

Understanding the spatial relationship of one artery to another is also helpful in properly identifying the intracranial arteries. Using the key reference signal, the terminal ICA (t-ICA) bifurcation as a guide, the locations of the intracranial arteries are found from the transtemporal window with more technical ease. Without using the relationship of one Doppler signal to another, identification of a signal as a particular artery becomes difficult.

Artery Traceability

The operator should "trace" the anatomic route of an artery in stepwise fashion by increasing/decreasing the depth setting of the sample volume. The ability to ultrasonically trace an artery within an expected depth range is important for proper identification, integrating blood flow direction and velocity as previously mentioned. Remember the rule "go with the flow", and try not to lose the signal while changing sample volume depths. Following the Doppler signals within the expected depth ranges is especially helpful for beginners when distinguishing the middle cerebral artery (30-67 mm) from the posterior cerebral artery (55-75 mm) from the transtemporal window.

Compression/Vibration Maneuvers

In most cases, proper identification of intracranial arteries does not require compression/oscillation of the common carotid artery (CCA). There are times, however, when compression maneuvers are useful in the identification of an intracranialartery and in the assessment of collateral pathways. If the operator believes common carotid artery compression is necessary, once again the importance of experienced personnel and selecting an artery free of significant disease cannot be overstated. Such information can be obtained easily by carotid duplex imaging.

If a compression maneuver is performed, the intracranial velocity signal may: 1) not change, 2) diminish, 3) disappear, 4) augment, or 5) change direction (reverse or alternating).

Normal Values

A number of investigators have studied and reported their findings in normal volunteers and from patients without neurological deficit at the time of the study and with unremarkable carotid duplex and TCD examinations.[1-10] When reviewing this literature, it is important to be aware of how the velocity measurements are reported. Most published TCD data are in velocities (centimeters/second; cm/sec), and that is the currently accepted format. Earlier publications reported values in frequencies (kiloHertz; kHz). To compare TCD values measured in frequency to those reported in velocity for transducers with an emitting frequency of 2 MHz, the formula $v = 0.039f$ can be used [v=velocity (cm/sec), f= Doppler frequency shift (Hz)]. It is also important to note if the numbers reported are the mean, peak systolic or end diastolic values.

It is customary to assume a zero degree angle when performing TCD examinations because the exact angle between the ultrasound beam and the intracranial arteries is unknown. The anatomic relationship between the intracranial arteries and the TCD windows produces actual transducer-artery angles somewhere between 0 and 30 degrees. For this range of transducer angles, the maximum error should be less than 15%.[1,11]

Different investigators have reported similar velocities for the same vessels demonstrating good interobserver agreement (Table 5-2). Mean velocity (time-averaged peak) are usually reported for TCD examinations since this parameter is less affected by changes of central cardiovascular factors (heart rate, peripheral resistance, etc.) than systolic or diastolic values[11], thereby diminishing inter-individual variations.[2,13]

Table 5-2. Intracranial arterial velocities by different investigators

	Mean Velocity (cm/sec)			
1st Author	MCA	ACA	PCA	Basilar
Aaslid	62 ± 12	51 ± 12	44 ±11	-
DeWitt	62 ± 12	52 ± 12	42 ± 10	42 ± 10
Grolimund	57 ± 15	49 ± 15	37 ± 10	-
Harders	65 ± 17	50 ± 13	40 ± 9	39 ± 9
Hennerici	58 ± 12	53 ± 11	37 ± 10	-
Lindegaard	67 ± 7	48 ± 5	42 ± 6	-
Ringelstein	55 ± 12	50 ± 11	39 ±10	41 ± 10
Russo	65 ± 13	48 ± 20	35 ±18	45 ± 10
Zanette	56 ± 12	50 ± 10	43 ± 7	-
Sorteberg	73 ± 11	58 ± 9	43 ± 10	-

Intracranial arterial velocities vary depending upon the age of the patient (Table 5-3). When performing a TCD examination, the operator and interpreter must be cognizant of the velocity changes expected with the patient's age.

Table 5-3. Intracranial arterial velocities by age

	Mean velocity (cm/sec)			
Age (yrs)	MCA	ACA	PCA	Basilar
10-29	70 ± 16	61 ± 15	55 ± 9	46 ± 11
30-49	57 ± 11	48 ± 7	42 ± 9	38 ± 9
50-59	51 ± 10	46 ± 9	39 ± 9	32 ± 7
60-70	41 ± 7	38 ± 6	36 ± 8	32 ± 7

Differences between intracranial arterial velocities are more important than the absolute values recorded from an individual.

General observations of the mean velocities in the intracranial arteries are: 1) the velocities are highest in the middle cerebral artery (MCA), 2) if an anterior cerebral artery (ACA) velocity is more than 25% greater than the MCA velocity, the ACA may be hypoplastic, stenotic, serving as a collateral vessel, or there may be a MCA distribution infarction, and 3) the velocities in the anterior circulation are higher than the posterior circulation.

Velocity Ratios

Evaluation of numerous inter-arterial ratios has failed to provide clinically useful information, with the exception of the ACA/MCA, MCA/ICA (cervical) ratio, and BA/VA ratios. As mentioned above, an ACA/MCA ratio greater than 1.2 is indicative of a pathologic situation present with the ACA (hypoplastic, stenosis, collateral channel), or of a MCA branch occlusion or a MCA distribution infarction.[14-16]

The MCA/ICA (cervical) ratio, the hemispheric index, or Lindegaard ratio, has been used to determine if changes in the MCA velocity are due to stenosis or volume flow,[17,18] thereby improving the diagnosis of vasospasm in patients with subarachnoid hemorrhage.[17] The normal range of this ratio has been reported to be from 1.1 - 3.0, with a mean of 1.8.[1,5,8]

Recently, Soustiel and colleagues have described a ratio of the basilar artery (BA) velocity to the velocity of the extracranial vertebral artery (EVA) that can be used to identify patients with hyperemic velocity increase as opposed to basilar artery vasospasm following subarachnoid hemorrhage.[19] In this study, a BA/EVA ratio >2.0 was associated with basilar artery vasospasm.

Side To Side Asymmetry

In the asymptomatic adult, side-to-side asymmetry should be minimal. The difference between sides has been reported to be less than 30% for normal vessels and undisturbed anatomy of the circle of Willis.[2,4,5,8] Small differences generally do not indicate an underlying pathological condition. If a side-to-side difference is noted during the TCD examination, try repeating the study on the side with the lower velocity. The operator must be certain that the best ultrasonic window was used on each side of the patient. Often by repeating the TCD study and modifying the transducer-to-artery angle, the side-to-side differences found on the initial examination can be reduced. If side-to-side differences occur, they should not be considered abnormal unless they exceed 30%. Additionally, it may be difficult to interpret marked asymmetries in the posterior cerebral and intracranial vertebral arteries due to variable anatomy and/or hypoplasia that often affect these vessels.

Observer Variability

Various technical factors, including the operator, can contribute to TCD measurement variability. In a study of 15 healthy volunteers, Maeda and colleagues demonstrated inter and intraobserver variability.[20] In this study, there were no significant changes in mean blood pressure and end-expiratory carbon dioxide partial pressure during repeated measurements. The correlation coefficients for the middle cerebral artery (MCA) and the basilar artery (BA) for the same examiner performing the examination on the same day were r=0.95 and r=0.83, respectively. Those values dropped to r=0.84 and r=0.69 when a repeated examination was performed by the same examiner on a different day (average 22 days apart). Interobserver variability was reported as having a correlation coefficient of r=0.90 for the MCA and r=0.78 for the BA.

The authors attribute the size of the ultrasound window and the possibility of different angles of insonation as the major source of the variance.

Totaro and colleagues[21] evaluated 36 patients with a mean age of 48 $\pm$ 16 years. Three measurements were made by the same examiner on each patient with a time interval of one hour between the first and second examinations, and approximately 24 hours between the first and third TCD examinations. The reproducibility of the velocities in the MCA, AVA, PCA and the BA were evaluated, and there was good reproducibility for all arteries between the first and second (r=0.78-0.96) and the first and third examinations (r=0.86-0.97).

Other studies have also reported similar findings.[5,22] The data provided by these studies indicate that day-to-day differences found by the same examiner do not exceed 20%. If a patient is being sequentially followed with TCD, however, these measurement limitations must be considered. Caution must also be advised when trying to interpret small velocity changes as real blood flow changes and not simply due to observer variability.

Pulsatility And Resistance Indices

The pulsatility index (P.I.) was first described by Gosling and colleagues in an attempt to quantify Doppler waveforms during the evaluation of lower extremity arterial disease.[23] Although most equipment automatically calculates the P.I. with each display sweep, it can be calculated from the following formula:

$$P.I. = \frac{Vs - Vd}{Vm}$$

Where Vs is the peak systolic velocity, Vd is the end diastolic velocity and Vm is the mean velocity.

When using the P.I., the resistance that is encountered with each cardiac cycle is considered. For example, damped blood flow distal to an obstruction will have a decreased P.I. (diastolic velocity greater than 50-60% of peak systolic). Doppler signals obtained proximal to a high resistance (i.e. increased intracranial pressure), however, will have an increased P.I. (pulsatile spectral waveform). The P.I. in the MCA is normally in the range of 0.5 - 1.1. In a study evaluating the variability in normal individuals, Sorteberg and colleagues found the P.I. to vary between 0.69 $\pm$ 0.11 and 0.71 $\pm$ 0.13 for the MCA, ACA, PCA, and there were no significant (<20%) side-to-side or day-to-day differences.[5]

Systemic cardiovascular characteristics (i.e. heart rate, blood pressure, etc.) may vary significantly between individuals, so the P.I. will also be variable. It is particularly affected by chronic hypertension and in these, often-older patients; it may be found as high as 1.2-1.8 in the MCA's with normal diameters.

In an attempt to correct for individual differences in input P.I., and to unmask potential arterial lesions in segments that are not directly assessable by ultrasound, Lindegaard and colleagues developed the pulsatility transmission index (PTI).[24] The PTI is the P.I. for the MCA expressed as percentage of the P.I. from a reference basal cerebral artery (PTI=P.I. (MCA) /P.I. (reference artery) x 100). The PTI is dependent on normal inflow conditions into the reference artery.

The resistance index (R.I.) was described by Pourcelot as another mathematical measure used to evaluate the resistance of the vascular bed. The pulsatility index, however, is the parameter more widely used for TCD examinations. Like the pulsatility index, an increased R.I. reflects increased distal vascular resistance. The resistance index is calculated by using the following formula:

$$RI = \frac{\text{peak systolic velocity - end diastolic velocity}}{\text{peak systolic velocity}}$$

It is important to remember that a good quality Doppler spectral waveform is necessary for the TCD equipment to accurately calculate the indices of pulsatility, since the values are derived from the maximum velocity envelope.

Spectral Broadening

Spectral broadening is observed in most TCD examinations. The Doppler sample volume size is usually larger than the intracranial arteries. In fact, the sample volume of 10 mm exceeds the entire cross-sectional lumen of an intracranial artery and includes bifurcations and small arterial branches. Therefore, even though historically spectral broadening was used as a diagnostic criterion for moderate degrees of stenosis in the extracranial carotid arteries, it is not helpful in refining the TCD interpretation.

Bruits and Musical Murmurs

Vibrations of anatomic structures transversed by the ultrasound beam cause phase shifts in the reflected echoes and modulate the received signal. The phase-modulated signals from vibrations are displayed symmetrically around the baseline. This phenomenon is always associated with increased intracranial velocities. Intracranial bruits appear as low frequency enhancement of the Doppler spectral waveform near the baseline. Intracranial musical murmurs have also been described during TCD examinations.[24] Musical murmurs appear as narrow bands symmetrical and parallel to the baseline, and have been described as sounding like the cooing of a bird.

Physiologic Factors

Age. TCD velocities are affected by the age of the patient. Several investigators have found lower intracranial arterial velocities with increasing age.[2,3,6-8,22,26] The downward trend in intracranial arterial velocities with increasing age may be multifactorial, but primarily results from changes in cardiac output and corresponds to an age-related decrease in cerebral blood flow (CBF). Dilative arteriopathy also occurs with age and could play a role in the lower velocities. The diameter differences alone, however, cannot explain the decreased CBF and, therefore, is not the primary explanation for the decreases in velocities demonstrated with increasing age.

Gender. Penetration of the temporal bone with the ultrasound beam is usually more difficult in females than in males.[27,28] However, once intracranial Doppler signals are obtained, there does not appear to be major differences in the velocity readings because of the sex of the patient. Two studies, however, have demonstrated a slight increase (3-5%) of MCA velocity in females.[8,22] Vriens and colleagues reported that females demonstrated the increase in intracranial arterial mean velocities during the third, fourth, and fifth decades.[22] Possible explanations for these findings are that females have a lower hematocrit, the intracranial arteries may be smaller in diameter, and it has been shown that women have higher hemispheric CBF than men.[8] The small differences documented in the intracranial arterial velocities because of the sex of the patient needs further investigation.

Hematocrit. Hematocrit (Hct) is the percentage of red blood cells by volume in whole blood and is a major determinant of blood viscosity. Blood viscosity is an important factor influencing intracranial arterial blood flow velocity. Intracranial velocities increase in the presence of anemia (Hct < 30%) in order to maintain the delivery of adequate amounts of oxygen. If anemia is the etiology for the elevated velocities, then these changes should be detected in all of the intracranial arteries. Focal or localized velocity increases suggest a different etiology.

Brass and colleagues evaluated the effects of hematocrit on MCA velocity in 45 patients.[29] They found an inverse relationship of velocity with hematocrit and concluded that TCD examinations made in the presence of anemia may need correction. Ameriso and colleagues evaluated 42 healthy volunteers (age range 63-86 years) and found a significant inverse association between mean MCA velocity and both hematocrit ($p<0.02$) and fibrinogen concentration ($p<0.005$).[30] Additionally, we have observed generalized increases in intracranial arterial velocities in patients with decreased hematocrits. Since it may be a factor in determining the clinical significance of the TCD data, the patient's hematocrit is documented on the data collection form when possible. Although the effect of a low hematocrit on TCD velocities should be recognized, precise formulas to compensate for this physiologic variant are not available. This may make it difficult to identify an intracranial stenosis in a patient with a low hematocrit.

Fever. A fever increases cerebral blood flow by approximately 10% for every degree of increase in temperature. Performing TCD examinations when a patient has a fever will result in increased intracranial arterial velocities compared to their baseline velocities. If a patient has a fever, the patient's temperature should be documented or if possible, the outpatient examination should be rescheduled.

Hypoglycemia. Patients who are hypoglycemic will increase cerebral blood flow to increase delivery of glucose to the brain. This is usually not a factor when performing TCD examinations, unless the glucose is less than 40mg%.

Carbon Dioxide. Changes in arterial carbon dioxide (CO2) partial pressure have an effect on cerebral blood flow and intracranial arterial velocities (Figure 5-1 A, B, C). Huber and Hander demonstrated angiographically that the diameter of the large basal arteries remain constant during changes in pCO2.[31] Alteration of cerebral vascular resistance and changes in the TCD signals are due to changes at the level of the arteriolar channels. Markwalder demonstrated that TCD could be used to measure MCA velocity changes induced by end-expiratory pCO2 changes and described an exponential increase in velocity with increasing pCO2 between 15 or 17 and 55 mmHg.[32]

Hyperventilation [deficiency of CO2 = hypocapnia] causes a decrease in the MCA mean velocity and an increase in the P.I. Hypoventilation [excess CO_2 = hypercapnia] causes an increase in MCA velocity and a decrease in the P.I. This information suggests that generalized changes in intracranial arterial velocities caused by CO_2 reactivity must be taken into account when interpreting the TCD data.

Additionally, if a patient falls asleep during the TCD examination, there is an increase in CO_2 resulting in an increase of cerebral blood flow and increased intracranial blood flow velocities. On the other hand, if a patient is crying during the TCD examination, there is a decrease in CO_2 resulting in a decrease in cerebral blood flow and a decrease in the intracranial arterial velocities. If a patient is sleeping or crying, this should be documented or if possible, the examination should be rescheduled.

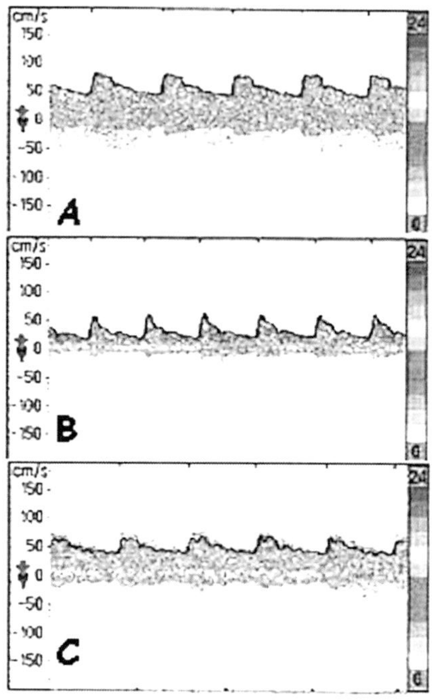

Figure 5-1. A MCA Doppler signal with: A) Normal breathing, B) Hyperventilation, and C) Breath holding.

Heart Rate/Cardiac Output/Blood Pressure. Intracranial arterial velocities are also a reflection of an individual's heart rate. Most experienced TCD examiners caution against taking a TCD reading if the patient is yawning, agitated, experiencing pain, or if there is any other reason causing a change in the heart rate. Any cardiac arrhythmia will be reflected in the TCD recording. If there is any question concerning a change in the patient's heart rate, then several display sweeps should be obtained before relying on the calculations. To compensate for extreme cases of bradycardia or tachycardia, the operator may need to adjust the instrument's display sweep time (Figure 5-2 A, B, C).

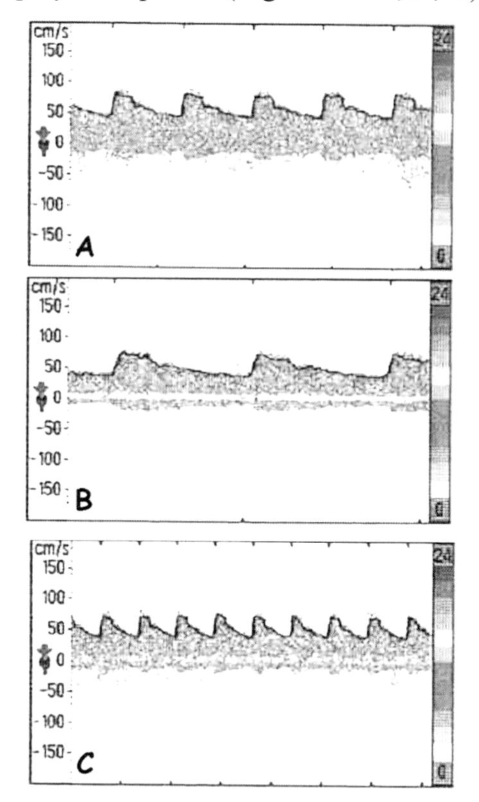

Figure 5-2. Different display sweep times: A) 4 seconds, B) 2 seconds, and C) 7 seconds.

Changes due to cardiac output not associated with hemodilution have little effect on CBF if autoregulation is intact.[33] This suggests that TCD velocities should be relatively independent of small changes in cardiac output. However, in severe cases of decreased cardiac output, cerebral blood flow may decrease resulting in decreased intracranial arterial velocities. Data on the relationship between cardiac output and intracranial arterial velocities are limited, and further investigation in this area is needed.

When there are changes in blood pressure, the cerebral arterioles respond to maintain a constant volume of cerebral blood flow (autoregulation). An increase in blood pressure causes the arterioles to constrict, increasing the resistance to flow, maintaining constant blood flow. In adults, minor changes in blood pressure will not affect the cerebral blood flow. Blood pressure has to be severely increased or decreased so that autoregulation cannot compensate, and there is a rise (hypertension) or fall (hypotension) in cerebral blood flow.

Brain Activity. TCD studies have shown an increase in PCA velocity in response to visual stimulation.[34] Additionally, increases in metabolic activity and regional CBF have been demonstrated with verbal, spatial, and/or manual tasks. Droste and colleagues reported experiments demonstrating MCA velocity increases ranging from 1.6% to 10.6% in 70 volunteers while performing right and left hemispheric tasks.[35] This increase in velocity was transient, but persisted for several seconds after the completion of the task. Kelley et al. evaluated the intracranial arterial velocities in 21 volunteers who performed mental arithmetic tasks and who played a commercially available video game.[36] Throughout the testing period, all subjects remained physiologically stable (pulse rate, blood pressure, PCO_2, etc.). A global increase in intracranial velocities was documented in the volunteers during task performance. Rihs and colleagues simultaneously evaluated MCAs bilaterally in fourteen healthy right-handed volunteers performing cognitive tasks.[37] Measuring bilateral MCA velocities simultaneously during the tasks helped to identify hemispheric dominance. A velocity shift (increase) to the left was demonstrated during language tasks, and during visuospatial tasks, there was a documented MCA velocity shift to the right side.

Velocity changes reported during cognitive activity should not cause a significant error when interpreting routine TCD examinations. The effects of inadvertent activation on intracranial arterial velocities are usually small, brief, and often bilateral. However, recognition of these changes must be considered when performing studies evaluating brain activity.[38] Using TCD to measure cerebral activation may lead to the development of an index for cerebral responsiveness to stimulation, or neuronal-vascular coupling that may assist in the diagnosis of vascular-related dementia in the future.

Limitations

There are several technical limitations when performing TCD examinations [Table 5-4]. Although all ultrasound studies are operator dependent, experience is the key factor when trying to obtain reliable, consistent TCD examinations. Operator experience will minimize errors associated with finding good temporal windows, arterial misidentification, and improper instrument control settings. Other problems such as anatomic variations, an unknown transducer-artery angle, distal branch disease, etc. that are inherent to the technique cannot be alleviated by the operator. Knowledge of the technique's limitations is important and should reduce errors associated with the interpretation of the TCD results.

TCD Interpretation

Many parameters are involved in the accurate interpretation of the TCD data. General interpretation guidelines are listed in Table 5-5. Each patient, however, must be considered individually because of the variety of physiologic factors that affect the intracranial arterial hemodynamics. The parameters that affect the intracranial velocities proximal to the circle of Willis are the patient's age, the location and extent of the extracranial obstruction, cardiac output, and hematocrit. At the level of the cerebral basal arteries are the vessel's diameter, blood viscosity, and turbulence. The parameters that affect the velocities distal to the circle of Willis are intracranial arteriovenous malformations (AVMs), cerebral infarction, increased intracranial pressure, and change in pCO_2.

Table 5-4. Limitations of the TCD examination

- Operator experience
- Absent or poor transtemporal windows
- Patient movement
- Anatomic variations
- Unknown transducer-to-artery Doppler angle
- Improper instrument control setting
- Arterial misidentification
- Displacement of arteries by an intracranial mass
- Misinterpretation of collateral channels or vasospasm as a stenosis
- Distal branch disease

Table 5-5. TCD interpretation guidelines

- Compare Doppler spectral waveforms (mean velocity) from the anterior and posterior circulation, and from the right and left sides
- Notice the Doppler spectral waveform configuration (pulsatility index, upstroke time)
- Consider disease in the patient's extracranial carotid and vertebral arterial systems
- Consider the patient's age, hematocrit, etc.
- Understand the limitations of the technique

The most useful TCD results are from comparing velocities from different sample volume depths from the same artery, and from comparing the velocities from the different arteries within an individual. Bilateral symmetric disease may be difficult to diagnose by TCD. Correct identification of the intracranial arteries, knowledge of the normal velocity ranges, familiarity of the technique's limitations, and how cerebral hemodynamics may be affected by different physiologic parameters are essential for the accurate interpretation of TCD examinations.

References

1. Aaslid R, Markwalder T-M, Nornes H. Noninvasive transcranial Doppler ultrasound recording of flow velocity in basal cerebral arteries. J Neurosurg 1982; 57:769-774.
2. Hennerici M, Rautenberg W, Sitzer G, Schwartz A. Transcranial Doppler ultrasound for the assessment of intracranial arterial flow velocity - Part 1. Examination technique and normal values. Surg Neurol 1987;27:439-448.
3. Ringelstein EB. A practical guide to transcranial Doppler sonography. In: Weinberger J (Ed): Noninvasive imaging of cerebrovasular disease. New York: A. Liss Publishers, 1989:75-121.
4. Zanette EM, Fieschi C, Bozzao L, et al. Comparison of cerebral angiography and transcranial Doppler sonography in acute stroke. Stroke 1989;20:899-903.
5. Sorteberg W, Langmoen IA, Lindegaard K-F, Nornes H. Side-to-side differences and day-to-day variations of transcranial Doppler parameters in normal subjects. J Ultrasound Med 1990;9:403-409.
6. Arnolds BJ, von Reutern G-M. Transcranial Doppler sonography. Examination technique and normal reference values. Ultrasound in Med & Biol 1986;12(2): 115-123.

7. Harders A. Neurosurgical Applications of transcranial Doppler Sonography. Normal Values. New York: Springer-Verlag,1986: 24-26.

8. Grolimund P, Seiler RW. Age dependence of the flow velocity in the basal cerebral arteries - A transcranial Doppler ultrasound study. Ultrasound in Med & Biol 1988;14 (3):191-198.

9. Russo G, Profeta G, Acamporas S, et al. Transcranial Doppler ultrasound examination technique and normal reference values. J Neurosur Sci 1986;30:97-102.

10. Dewitt LD, Wechsler LR. Transcranial Doppler. Stroke 1988;19:915-921.

11. Aaslid R. The Doppler principle applied to measurement of blood flow velocity in cerebral arteries. In Aaslid R (ed): Transcranial Doppler Sonography. New York: Springer-Verlag, Chapter 3, 1986:22-38.

12. Aaslid R. Transcranial Doppler examination techniques. In Aaslid R (ed). Transcranial Doppler Sonography. New York: Springer-Verlag, Chapter 4, 1986:39-59.

13. Caplan LR, Brass LM, DeWitt LD, et al. Transcranial Doppler ultrasound: present status. Neurology 1990; 40:696-700.

14. Mattle H, Grolimund P, Huber P, et al. Transcranial Doppler sonographic findings in middle cerebral artery disease. Arch Neurol 1988;45:289-295.

15. Adams RJ, Nichols FT, Hess DC, et al. Transcranial Doppler: Clinical utility in the evaluation of patients with atherosclerotic cerebrovascular disease. Neurology 1989;39 (suppl 1):304.

16. Grolimund P, Seiler RW, Aaslid R, et al. Evaluation of cerebrovascular disease by combined extracranial and transcranial Doppler Sonography experience in 1,309 patients. Stroke 1987;18:1018-1024.

17. Lindegaard K-F, Nornes H, Bakke SJ, et al. Cerebral vasospasm diagnosis by means of angiography and blood flow velocity measurements. Acta Neurochir 1989;100:12-24.

18. Aaslid R, Huber P, Nornes H. A transcranial Doppler method in the evaluation of cerebrovascular vasospasm. Neuroradiology 1986; 28:11-16.

19. Soustiel JF, Shik V, Shreiber R, et. al. Basilar vasospasm diagnosis: investigation of a modified "Lindegaard Index" based on imaging studies and blood velocity measurements of the basilar artery. Stroke 2002;33:72-77.

20. Maeda H, Etani H, Handa N, et al. A validation study on the reproducibility of transcranial Doppler velocimetry. Ultrasound Med Biol 1990;16:9-14.

21. Totaro R, Marini C, Cannarsa C, Prencipe M. Reproducibility of transcranial Doppler sonography: a validation study. Ultrasound Med Biol 1992;18:173-177.

22. Vriens EM, Kraaier V, Musbach M, et al. Transcranial pulsed Doppler measurements of blood velocity in the middle cerebral artery: reference values at rest and during hyperventilation in healthy volunteers in relation to age and sex. Ultrasound Med Biol 1989;15:1-8.

23. Gosling RG, Dunbar G, King DH, et al. The quantitative analysis of occlusive peripheral arterial disease by a non-intrusive ultrasonic technique. Angiology 1971;22:52-55.

24. Lindegaard K-F, Bakke SJ, Grolimund P, et al. Assessment of intracranial hemodynamics in carotid artery disease by transcranial Doppler ultrasound. J Neurosurg 1985;63:890-898.

25. Aaslid R, Nornes H. Musical murmurs in human cerebral arteries after subarachnoid hemorrhage. J Neurosurg 1984;60:32-36.

26. Ringelstein EB, Kahlscheuer B, Niggemeyer E, Otis SM. Transcranial Doppler sonography: Anatomical landmarks and normal velocity values. Ultrasound in Med & Biol 1990;16:745-761.

27. Halsey JH. Effect of emitted power on waveform intensity in transcranial Doppler. Stroke 1990;21:1573-1578.

28. Halsey JH. Response: Letter to the editor. Stroke 1991;22:533-534.

29. Brass LM, Pavlakis SG, DeVivo D, et al. Transcranial Doppler measurements of the middle cerebral artery. Effect of hematocrit. Stroke 1988; 19:1466-1469.

30. Ameriso SF, Paganini-Hill A, Meiselman HJ, Fisher M. Correlates of middle cerebral artery blood velocity in the elderly. Stroke 1990;21:1579-1583.

31. Huber P, Handa J. Effect of contrast material, hypercapnia, hyperventilation, hypertonic glucose and papaverine on the diameter of the cerebral arteries. Angiographic Determination In Man. Invest Radiol 1967;2:17-32.

32. Markwalder T-M, Grolimund P, Seiler RW, et al. Dependency of blood flow velocity in the middle cerebral artery on end-tidal carbon dioxide partial pressure - A transcranial ultrasound Doppler study. J Cerebral Blood Flow and Metabolism 1984;4:368-372.

33. Bouma GJ, Muizelaar JP. Relationship between cardiac output and cerebral blood flow in patients with intact and with impaired autoregulation. J Neurosurg 1990;73:368-374.

34. Aaslid R. Visually evoked dynamic blood flow response of the human cerebral circulation. Stroke 1987;18: 771-775.

35. Droste DW, Harders AG, Rastogi E. A transcranial Doppler study of blood flow velocity in the middle cerebral arteries performed at rest and during mental activities. Stroke 1989;20: 1005-1011.

36. Kelly RE, Chang JY, Scheinman NJ, et al. Transcranial Doppler assessment of cerebral blood flow velocity during cognitive tasks. Stroke 1992;23:9-14.

37. Rihs F, Gutbrod K, Gutbrod B, et al. Determination of cognitive hemispheric dominance by "stereo" transcranial Doppler sonography. Stroke 1995;26:70-73.

38. Klingelhofer J, Sander D. Transcranial Doppler ultrasonography monitoring during cognitive testing. In: Tegeler CH, Babikian VL, Gomez CR (eds): Neurosonology. St. Louis: Mosby; Chapter 18, 1996:200-213.

Chapter 6
Clinical Applications

The clinical applications (Table 6-1) of transcranial Doppler (TCD) have expanded since the technique's introduction in 1982. Investigators find that information about intracranial arterial hemodynamics is valuable in many different clinical settings.

This chapter is an introductory description of: 1) the variety of clinical applications for TCD examinations, 2) the technical nuances of the TCD examination associated with those applications, and 3) the interpretation criteria used for the various applications.

Table 6-1. Clinical applications of TCD

- Diagnosis of intracranial vascular disease.
- Monitoring vasospasm in subarachnoid hemorrhage.
- Screening of children with sickle cell disease.
- Assessment of intracranial collateral pathways.
- Evaluation of the hemodynamic effects of extracranial occlusive disease on intracranial blood flow.
- Intraoperative monitoring.
- Detection of cerebral emboli.
- Monitoring evolution of cerebral circulatory arrest.
- Documentation of subclavian steal.
- Evaluation of the vertebrobasilar system.
- Detection of feeders of arteriovenous malformations (AVMs).
- Monitoring anticoagulation regimens or thrombolytic therapy.
- Monitoring during neuroradiologic interventions.
- Testing of functional reserve.
- Monitoring after head trauma.

Diagnosis of intracranial disease

The ability to detect intracranial arterial stenosis, occlusion, and aneurysms is a new and potentially important addition to the noninvasive cerebrovascular examination. However, to accurately assess the intracranial vasculature, one must be cognizant of the hemodynamic changes associated with intracranial (and extracranial) disease.

Intracranial arterial stenoses cause characteristic alterations in the Doppler spectral waveform that include focal increases in velocity (Figure 6-1), local turbulence, and a post-stenotic drop in velocity. These changes associated with a stenosis occur assuming that volume flow is maintained. Stenoses may also produce low frequency enhancement around the baseline (bruit), or band shaped enhancements symmetrical and parallel to the baseline (musical murmur) as well as compensatory flow velocity increase in a branching vessel.

A focal stenosis greater than 50% diameter reduction usually will be detected by TCD since it causes at least a "doubling" of the velocity compared to a normal segment. Absolute velocity criteria for the diagnosis of an intracranial arterial stenosis are not reliable, due to the many velocity alterations caused by nonvascular variables (age, hematocrit, etc). A mean velocity of 80 cm/sec in the (MCA), the anterior cerebral artery (ACA), the posterior cerebral artery (PCA), or the terminal internal carotid artery (t-ICA) is the threshold causing concern while 100 cm/sec is more predictive of a ≥ 50% MCA stenosis. The mean velocity at which suspicion is raised for a stenosis in the vertebrobasilar system is 70 cm/sec. Additionally, an intracranial arterial stenosis should be suspected when the

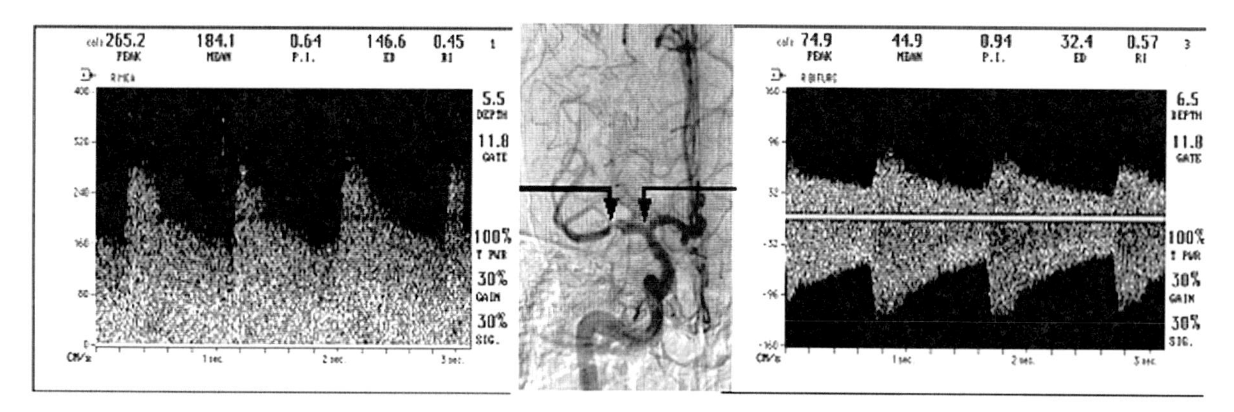

Figure 6-1. A high grade stenosis of the middle cerebral artery. The mean velocity was 184 cm/sec. at the site of the arterial narrowing (55mm). The mean velocity was 45 cm/sec. in the proximal MCA (65mm).

normal hierarchy of velocities is disrupted (i.e. MCA>ACA>PCA>BA >VA).

Since absolute velocities are inaccurate, most investigators agree that a focal velocity increase of ≥ 25% should raise suspicion of an arterial narrowing. Additionally, a focal stenosis is usually accompanied by turbulence. Frequent Doppler sampling of the arteries (every 2 to 5 mm) is important to localize Doppler signal changes associated with a stenosis. Intracranial stenoses are most commonly found in the carotid siphon, the terminal ICA bifurcation, and in the MCA. The incidence of an isolated intracranial stenosis in the anterior or posterior cerebral arteries is low. The status of the cerebral tissue that is perfused by the vessel can also have a significant impact on its intracranial velocity profiles. Patients with the stenosis of the M1 segment of the without acute infarction demonstrate an increased MCA velocity. However, the same patient with an acute or evolving cerebral infarction may have diminished MCA velocity, depending on the size and location of the infarct, and because of the decreased perfusion (demand) to the infarcted area.

TCD is limited in its ability to reliably identify intracranial arterial occlusion. This limitation arises from inadequate transtemporal windows, anatomic variability, and congenital aplasia or severe hypoplasia of the other intracranial arteries.

Middle cerebral artery occlusion (Figure 6-2) is suspected when a MCA Doppler signal is absent and good quality Doppler signals are obtained from the uninvolved ipsilateral intracranial arteries (t-ICA, ACA, PCA). Locating the other ipsilateral arteries demonstrates that an adequate transtemporal window exists. Important technical features when evaluating a patient for a MCA occlusion are decreasing the depth of the sample volume after locating the terminal internal-ICA bifurcation, changing the transducer's angle, adjusting the Doppler and color Doppler gain settings, and lowering the color PRF. Identifying the contralateral MCA in its expected anatomic location reduces the chance of aberrant anatomy. An increase in the ipsilateral anterior cerebral artery velocity due to perfusion through leptomeningeal collaterals is considered corroborating evidence for a MCA occlusion.[1] Patients with acute cerebral infarcts with MCA occlusion may demonstrate recanalization if followed with serial TCD examinations, therefore, the TCD results may vary depending on the timing of the examination from the cerebral

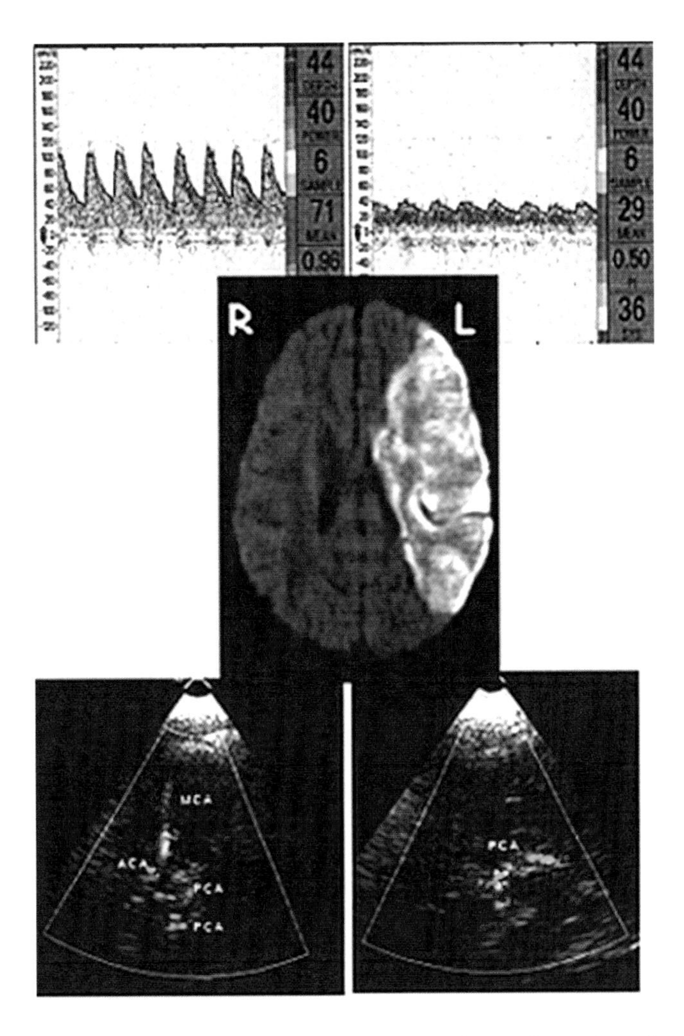

Figure 6-2. Left MCA occlusion. The TCD examination was performed one day after the event. The MCA Doppler signal is significantly decreased on the left side compared to the right MCA Doppler signal. The TCDI of the left side demonstrated a patent posterior circulation and the absence of a color Doppler signal from the anterior circulation.

event. Information regarding the sensitivity and specificity of TCD in the diagnosis of intracranial stenoses and occlusion is limited.[1-13] The lack of reliable data is due to the overall low incidence of intracranial disease and the small number of patients who have good quality intracranial arteriograms after TCD identifies disease. The sensitivity of TCD varies depending upon the artery insonated and the experience of the TCD operator. The sensitivity for diagnosing a MCA stenosis ranges from 73-94%.

de Bray and colleagues reported the sensitivity of identifying a MCA stenosis by TCD depended upon the diameter reduction of the stenosis.[6] Seventy-five percent (9/12) of the patients with a stenosis greater than 50% were identified by TCD, whereas only one of four patients with a lesser stenosis was identified in this study.

Arenillas and colleagues followed the progression of MCA stenoses with TCD.[14] The patients had the intracranial stenosis identified by TCD and confirmed by arteriography, and they were regularly followed with TCD for a median follow-up of 26.6 months. The progression of the MCA stenosis documented by TCD was independently associated with a new ipsilateral ischemic event (p=0.031), suggesting that TCD may be a useful tool to follow the progression of intracranial arterial lesions.

Data are limited regarding transcranial Doppler's sensitivity in the diagnosis of intracranial aneurysms. Harders reported that there was no change in the TCD spectral waveforms in more than 90 patients with small (<1cm) intracranial aneurysms.[15] In patients with larger intracranial aneurysms, however, changes in the waveforms were found that included a decrease in velocity, an increase in peripheral resistance, bruits, and multiple peaks during systole. There may also be an increase in velocity in the neck of the aneurysm, and varying degrees of velocity, pulsatility, and turbulence within the aneurysm depending on the location of the Doppler sample volume. And if an aneurysm compresses the adjacent artery, focal increases in velocity may also be observed.

The sensitivity of detecting a patent intracranial aneurysm using transcranial color Doppler imaging depends upon the aneurysm's location and size and has been reported to be from 0 to 85%.[16-19] In the most optimistic report, Baumgartner and colleagues identified 85% (23/27) of non-thrombosed aneurysms with a diameter of 6 to 25 mm.[16] Four non-thrombosed aneurysms were missed that had a mean diameter of 5 mm, and three thrombosed aneurysms were missed. One would not expect transcranial color Doppler imaging to identify thrombosed intracranial aneurysms due to the absence of blood flow. Martin and colleagues, using color Doppler imaging, were unable to detect any of the 11 known intracranial aneurysms in five patients.[17] In this study, all aneurysms had an angiographically determined diameter of ≤ 5 mm. Differentiation of a dilation versus color artifact is difficult, since the high color gain setting used during transcranial color Doppler imaging cause color spill over into the adjacent tissue. Additionally, during TCD imaging, vessel tortuousity or branching may be misdiagnosed as an aneurysm.

Wardlaw and Cannon identified 26 of 37 intracranial aneurysms using color power Doppler imaging.[19] In this exploratory study, the investigators found the following ultrasound features useful in the identification of intracranial aneurysms: 1) rounded color areas projecting from an artery that appear noncontinuous at both ends with an artery; 2) color flow appearing in an unexpected area; 3) a color area that is wider than the adjacent arteries; and 4) an area with greater expansion and contraction during the cardiac cycle compared to the adjacent artery. The ultrasound characteristics suggested by these investigators may be helpful in diagnosing intracranial aneurysms. However, the importance of proper instrument control settings cannot be over-emphasized.

Sources of error in the TCD diagnosis of intracranial disease are: 1) misinterpreting collateral channels or vasospasm as stenoses (vasospasm usually involves several arteries and the velocities change with time); 2) the technical limitations of evaluating distal branch disease (stenosis or occlusion); 3) the misinterpretation of a tortuous or displaced MCA (by hematoma or tumor) diagnosed as an occlusion; 4) anatomic variability (location, asymmetry, tortuousity), especially in the vertebrobasilar system; 5) technical difficulty in the evaluation of the distal basilar artery; 6) the location of cerebral aneurysms and if the aneurysm is small; and 7) poor quality arteriography leading to inaccurate correlations of the TCD results.

Effects Of Extracranial Occlusive Disease On Intracranial Perfusion

Extracranial occlusive disease can have a variable effect on intracranial arterial hemodynamics. Several factors (the diameter reduction and location of the stenosis, the patency of the collateral pathways, infarction, autoregulation, and so forth) affect intracranial arterial velocities. Since intracranial arterial velocities are not uniformly affected by extracranial disease, they cannot be used to reliably diagnose extracranial disease. Severe extracranial disease may result in decreased velocities, delayed systolic upstroke, and reduced pulsatility indices in the intracranial arteries ipsilateral to the disease. However, some patients may demonstrate normal intracranial arterial velocities even in the presence of significant extracranial disease.

Transcranial Doppler reveals intracranial arterial collateral patterns in patients with extracranial stenosis. Although the operator performs a standard TCD examination, s/he must be aware of the variable effect of extracranial disease on the intracranial arterial velocity profiles, and the potential collateral pathways that occur in response to extracranial disease.

An artery providing collateral circulation usually demonstrates an increased blood flow velocity. Unlike focal increases in velocity found in an arterial stenosis, collateral pathways contain diffuse velocity increases throughout the length of the artery. An artery providing collateral circulation must increase its flow velocity due to the increased blood flow demand.

The three main collateral pathways identified by TCD are: 1) the anterior communicating artery (ACoA) providing a channel from hemisphere to hemisphere; 2) the posterior communicating artery (PCoA) allowing blood to flow between the posterior and the anterior circulation; and 3) the ophthalmic artery (OA) providing a channel from the extracranial external carotid artery (ECA) to the intracranial internal carotid artery (ICA) through the orbit.

The most commonly found collateral pattern in response to significant extracranial carotid disease is via the anterior communicating artery (Figure 6-3). The ultrasound characteristics of this collateral pathway include: 1) an increase in the contralateral anterior cerebral artery velocity; 2) a turbulent Doppler signal with increased velocity at midline (due to high velocity flow through the small ACoA); and 3) reversal of blood flow in the ipsilateral ACA.

Collateral perfusion from the posterior to the anterior circulation, via increased blood flow through the posterior communicating artery (Figure 6-4) is the second pattern and is found most often when patients have significant bilateral extracranial carotid artery disease. When this collateral pathway is evoked the ipsilateral PCA will demonstrate increased velocity proximal to the origin of the PCoA and decreased velocity when the PCA is tracked distally.

The external carotid artery collateral pathway through the orbit is the third collateral pattern. It is documented by reversed blood flow direction in the ophthalmic artery carrying blood flow from the ECA to the intracranial ICA (Figure 6-5). In addition, the shape of the OA Doppler signal changes from a high to a low resistance signal because the blood flow in the artery is now supplying the brain.

Studies have shown good correlation of TCD and arteriography in the identification of collateral patterns.[5,20,21] Lindegaard and colleagues demonstrated a sensitivity of 94%

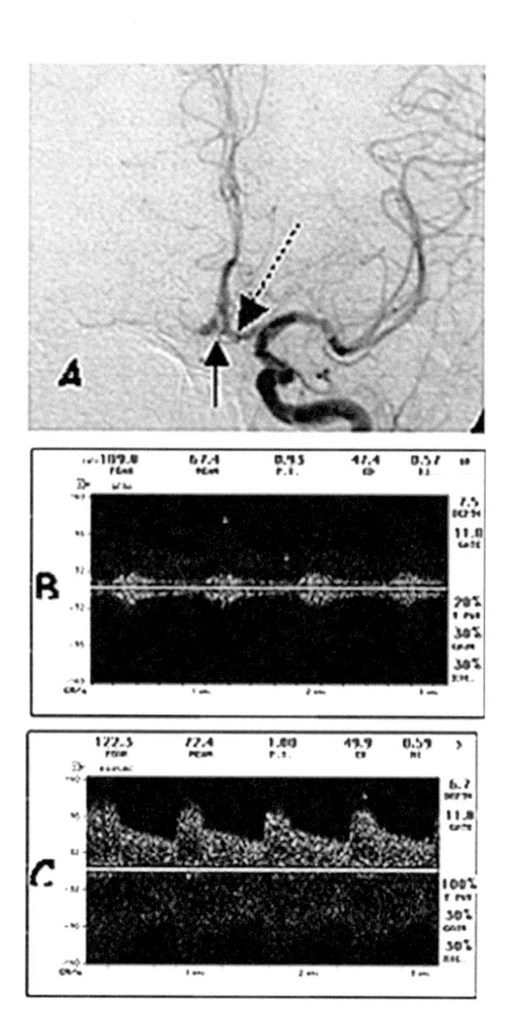

Figure 6-3. A) Left-to-right cross-filling via the anterior communicating artery (solid arrow). Dotted arrow points to the left ACA. B) The anterior cerebral artery mean velocity is elevated (67 cm/sec) on the right side and blood flow direction is reversed. C) The Doppler spectral waveform from the donor ACA near midline demonstrates elevated velocities (blood flow direction is away from the transducer).

(29/31) for the anterior communicating artery pathway and 87% (26/30) for the collateral pathway involving the posterior communicating artery.[20] Likewise, Grolimund and colleagues found the sensitivity for identifying the ACoA pathway to be 94% (16/17), the PCoA was 88% (7/8), and the ECA collateral pathway through the orbit was 89% (8/9).[5] A study of six medical centers however, reported a sensitivity of only 62% (18/29) for the ACoA and 100% (7/7) for OA collateral pathway.[21]

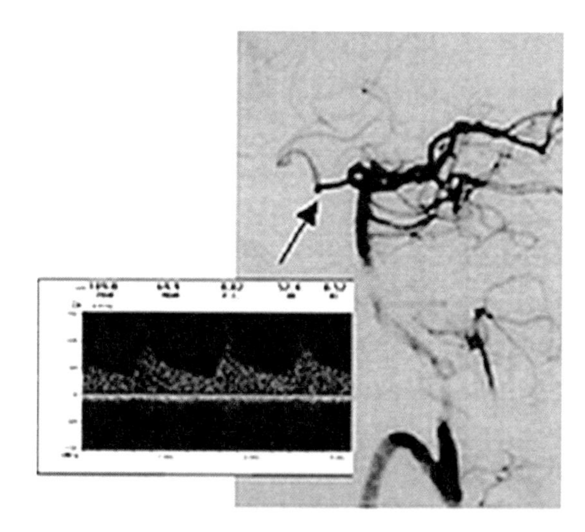

Figure 6-4. Collateral blood flow via the posterior communicating artery (arrow). Blood flow is from the posterior to the anterior circulation in this patient.

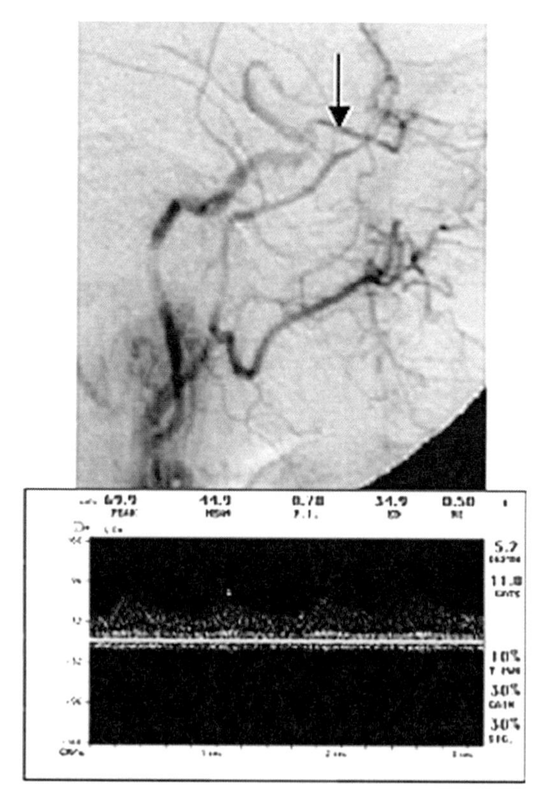

Figure 6-5. Reversed blood flow direction in the ophthalmic artery (arrow). Blood flow is away from the transducer (inverted waveform) and demonstrates a low resistance pattern because it is supplying blood to the brain.

A potential source of error in these correlative studies is that arteriography may not always demonstrate true physiologic conditions. Discrepancies between the TCD examination and arteriography may be due to the pressure of the contrast injection during the x-ray and, therefore, TCD may provide a more accurate indication of functional collateral blood flow then arteriography. Additionally, the posterior collateral is often difficult to identify, and represents a technical source of error during transcranial Doppler examinations.

Functional Reserve Testing

Cerebral blood flow (CBF) is maintained over a wide range of perfusion pressures or modulated by vasoconstriction and vasodilation of the arterioles. TCD offers a noninvasive means of evaluating whether extracranial carotid disease affects intracranial hemodynamics to the degree as to place the patient at risk for a low-flow mechanism for stroke.

When patients have exhausted their cerebrovascular reserve, the resistance arteries of the brain are maximally dilated and are unresponsive to any further vasodilator stimulus. Hypercapnia (excess carbon dioxide in blood) in this setting will not increase blood flow. When this occurs ischemic brain injury can result if perfusion pressure is further reduced. Identification of patients suffering severe hypoperfusion and who, therefore, may benefit from revascularization (carotid endarterectomy or perhaps extracranial-intracranial bypass) is based on the detection of an exhausted cerebrovascular reserve.[22-27]

To study whether the patient has reached a state where the cerebral circulation has been maximally dilated, a potent vasodilator (carbon dioxide [CO_2]) can be used to enhance CBF in both hemispheres. The CO_2 affects the peripheral vascular bed (distal cerebral arteries) and does not affect the diameters of the large basal arteries.[28] Since changes in velocity do not reflect diameter variation in the M1 segment, TCD monitoring of the middle cerebral artery is a reliable indicator of the collateral reserve capacity in patients.[29]

Ringelstein and colleagues evaluated the vasomotor reserve in forty healthy volunteers.[26] There was a mean MCA velocity increase of 52.5% during hypercapnia and a decrease of 35.3% during hypocapnia (deficiency of carbon dioxide). In the same study, forty patients with unilateral ICA occlusion, had a significantly lower vasomotor reactivity on the occluded side (45.2%) versus the non-occluded side (67.7%) [$p<0.0001$]. Additionally, the vasomotor reactivity was significantly lower in patients with symptomatic ICA occlusion than in asymptomatic patients (37.6% vs. 62.9%; $p<0.006$).

Park and colleagues used TCD to measure the autoregulatory response for the basilar artery in sixteen normal subjects. In this study, the investigators demonstrated that the autoregulatory index and the CO_2 reactivity values for the basilar artery to be similar to those for the middle cerebral artery.[178]

To evaluate the vasomotor reserve, patients are examined in the supine position. A mask is placed on the face and the patient breathes room air for a few minutes to record stable baseline velocities. The MCA velocities are recorded at a depth of 50 mm with patient breathing room air, breathing a mixture of 5% CO_2 with a balance of oxygen during maximum hypercapnia and hypocapnia. The end tidal (expired) carbon dioxide values are also monitored throughout the testing period. When monitoring patients for MCA velocity changes due to CO_2 reactivity, it is helpful to use a specially designed monitoring headpiece. The headpiece will hold the TCD transducer at the same angle, and the recorded changes accurately reflect those caused by increases in pCO_2. If the operator holds the transducer in place, it is important not to vary the transducer's angle. The operator can minimize inadvertent hand movements by being in a comfortable position at the patient's head, with the elbow of the examining arm resting on the examination table.

Markus and Harrison[30] compared a breath holding index (BHI) to estimate cerebrovascular reactivity to the techniques described by Ringelstein[26] and Bishop.[31] All three methods correlated significantly with the degree of stenosis in 23 patients.

The breath holding technique is a convenient screening method to assess carbon dioxide reactivity because it does not require administration of carbon dioxide. BHI is the simplest way of challenging vasomotor reactivity if the patient is compliant and capable of holding their breath for 30 seconds. This index is calculated by dividing the percent increase in mean velocity (MV) that occurs during breath-holding by the length of the time (30 seconds) that the patient holds their breath after normal inspiration. The formula to calculate the BHI is:

([MV-end – MV–rest/MV-rest] x 100)/30.

To perform the breath-holding test, the patient should be able to hold their breath voluntarily for at least 24 seconds, preferably 30 seconds. This may be difficult for some patients. The following suggestions may be useful to help the patient complete this test; 1) explain the test procedure and its importance in detail to the patient, 2) demonstrate to the patient that no major chest excursions should be made at the beginning and end of breath holding (major chest volume changes with forced breathing change intra-thoracic pressure and may affect velocity and flow pulsatility), 3) it is helpful to the patient to announce the time remaining at 10 seconds intervals after breath-holding has started (this helps the patient to be more confident that she or he can complete the test), and 4) before recording the value for the baseline mean velocity, wait about 4 seconds after the patient starts to breath (i.e. optimized signals).

BHI values of less than 0.69 are predictive of risk of stroke in patients with asymptomatic severe ICA stenoses and symptomatic occlusions.[32,33] This TCD test does not require any gas monitoring equipment or intravenous injections. Although subjectivity of patient effort and the unknowns of blood gas concentration make this test probably less reliable, it has been prospectively validated to predict clinical outcomes in patients with occlusive ICA disease. BHI may represent a screening test in the outpatient clinic to identify patients with impaired vasomotor reactivity.

Kleiser and Widder measured CO_2 reactivity in 85 patients with ICA occlusion (bilateral in 4 patients) to evaluate the risk of stroke.[34] Patients were categorized according to their CO_2 reactivity (sufficient, diminished, exhausted) and were prospectively followed for 38 $\pm$ 15 (mean $\pm$ SD) months. In the group with sufficient CO_2 reactivity, 8% (4/48) developed a transient ischemic attack (TIA) or prolonged reversible deficit; however, none had a stroke. In patients with a diminished or exhausted cerebrovascular reserve, 32% (12/37) developed an ipsilateral event, including a stroke in 8 and a TIA in 4 patients ($p<0.01$).

Vasospasm

Cerebral vasospasm (vaso-constriction of the intracerebral arteries) is a serious complication following subarachnoid hemorrhage (SAH), and is a significant cause of morbidity and mortality. The most common cause of SAH is leakage of blood from intracranial cerebral aneurysms into the subarachnoid space. Common sites for intracranial aneurysm formation are the anterior communicating artery, the middle cerebral artery, and the posterior cerebral artery. Early diagnosis and treatment reduces the devastating consequences of this disorder.

The hemodynamic effect of vasospasm produces an increase in blood flow velocity coupled with a pressure drop distal to the narrowed segment. Patients compensate for this and maintain cerebral blood flow through their collateral circulation and cerebral autoregulation. When there is increased intracranial pressure and/or the vasomotor reserve has been exhausted, cerebral blood flow can be reduced to critical levels resulting in ischemia or infarction.

Prior to TCD, arteriography was the only method to diagnose vasospasm. The arteriographic diagnosis of vasospasm is subjective, variable due to timing, difficult to measure, and demonstrates significant interobserver variability.[35] Arteriography is expensive and risky in patients with vasospasm and, therefore, is limited as a monitoring technique. The arterial narrowing produced by the spasm, however, causes an increase in blood flow velocity which can be quantified by TCD.[36-50] The evaluation of the vasospasm over time, and its response to treatment, can be monitored by TCD (Figure 6-6).

Since the increase in velocity detected by TCD often precedes the onset of neurologic deterioration and symptomatic vasospasm does not always occur on Day 7, TCD can be used to determine the correct timing for arteriography and intravascular intervention, or the need to continue or intensify pharmacologic intervention (triple H-therapy: hypertension-hemodilution-hypervolemia).[3]

Examinations are usually performed bedside in the intensive care unit (ICU). Prior to moving the TCD equipment to the ICU, it is beneficial to call the nurses and arrange a

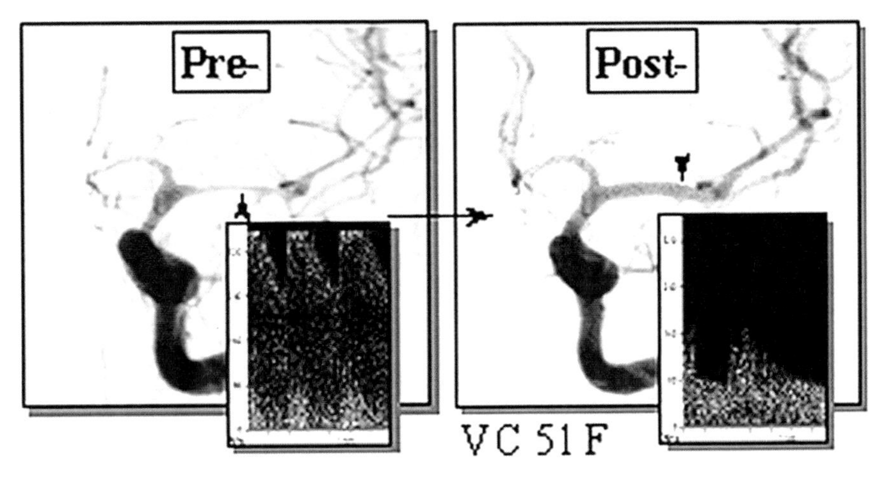

Figure 6-6. Pre and post angioplasty of the MCA in a 51 year old female with vasospasm. The mean velocity was 302 cm/sec prior to angioplasty and post-angioplasty the mean velocity decreased to 106 cm/sec.

convenient time to examine the patient. The important technical features when studying the patient with vasospasm associated with SAH are: 1) the operator must be properly positioned at the patient's bedside to make appropriate adjustments in transducer-to-artery angle; 2) the equipment is portable and there is a recording device; 3) a remote control is available to make adjustments to the TCD controls and the recording device (this will vary depending upon the type of equipment); 4) headphones are required because high (velocity) signals associated with vasospasm can be difficult to appreciate if there is extraneous background noise; 5) the precise location of the transtemporal window should be marked on the patient's skin, if possible, so that subsequent examinations can be performed from the same location, thereby ensuring the most reliable comparison; and 6) if possible, repeat evaluations should be performed by the same operator to eliminate interobserver variability.

In some patients, the surgical head dressing may need to be lifted or removed to obtain access to the transtemporal window. Sterile ultrasound gel is used if the transducer is placed near a wound. TCD recording is possible through a burr hole. However, the equipment's intensity level should be decreased since the bone no longer causes attenuation of the Doppler signal. TCD examinations in this group of patients can be challenging due to variable patient cooperation, changing cardiovascular and cerebral hemodynamic, and less than optimal testing conditions. Clip artifacts and a general hyperdynamic state of perfusion may mask localized segments of increased velocity.

Vasospasm is unusual the first two to three days following SAH. Therefore, a TCD examination during this pre-spastic period serves as a valuable baseline. It allows monitoring of the rate at which vasospasm develops, and provides a guide to future examinations since vessels in spasm are small and can be difficult to locate. Available arteriograms can be used to help locate the intracranial arteries and confirm TCD findings.

The TCD examination should be performed daily or every other day for two weeks, and the highest velocity obtained from each artery should be recorded. The frequency of the TCD examination is guided by the patient's clinical presentation, knowledge of risk factors for vasospasm, and the early clinical course. Although a complete TCD examination is preferred, it is not always possible in these patients. Additionally, a cervical ICA velocity signal is obtained at a depth of 45-55 mm (without angle adjustment) to calculate a hemispheric ratio. The frequency of follow-up studies will vary depending on clinical symptoms and the degree of vasospasm. It is useful to monitor the maximum mean velocity obtained for each intracranial artery since some patients with abnormal breathing patterns display periodic changes in velocities due to changes in pCO_2. The pCO2, hematocrit, and blood pressure should be recorded because these parameters may affect the intracranial arterial blood flow velocities. The time and the date of the examination is documented, and a graph plotting velocity versus time illustrates the time course of a patient's vasospasm. Following SAH, velocity increases begin to occur about day three, reach a maximum between days 7-12, and generally resolve at 2 to 3 weeks.

Middle cerebral artery mean velocities of 100-120 cm/sec correlate with mild vasospasm as demonstrated by arteriography.

Moderate vasospasm is defined by velocities in the 120-200 cm/sec range, and severe vasospasm is characterized by velocities exceeding 200 cm/sec. Mean velocities > 200 cm/sec indicate that the patient is at risk of reduced cerebral blood flow (CBF). A rapid increase (>25 cm/sec per day) in velocity in the first few days after the hemorrhage is associated with a poor prognosis.[37] Musical murmurs have been observed in patients being monitored for vasospasm, although their clinical relevance is uncertain.[45]

Lindegaard and colleagues use an MCA/ICA (distal extracranial ICA) mean velocity ratio to determine vasospasm.[48] This hemispheric ratio accounts for a possible increase in the flow volume. The ratio increases with severe spasm due to increased MCA velocity, and reduced blood flow volume in the ipsilateral extracranial ICA due to the increase in cerebral vascular resistance. The normal range for the MCA/ICA ratio is 1.7 ± 0.4. A MCA/ICA ratio >3 corresponds to MCA vasospasm, and a ratio >6 demonstrates severe vasospasm.

Recently, investigators have evaluated a ratio of the basilar artery (BA) velocity to the velocity of the extracranial vertebral artery (EVA) that can be used to identify patients with hyperemic velocity increase as opposed to basilar artery vasospasm following subarachnoid hemorrhage.[49,50] Soustiel and colleagues found a BA/EVA ratio >2.0 was associated with basilar artery vasospasm.[50] The sensitivity for diagnosing vasospasm by TCD depends on the skill of the operator, the presence of a ultrasound window, anatomic consistency, a good transducer-to-artery angle, the location and the severity of the vasospasm, the presence of proximal hemodynamically significant lesions, physiologic parameters (increased intracranial pressure, blood pressure fluctuations, pCO2 variations, hematocrit, etc.), the diagnostic criteria used, current medications, and the age and the cooperation of the patient. The sensitivity of detecting vasospasm of the MCA has been reported to be from 39 to 94% and the specificity from 85 to 100%.[40,42,46,51,52] Data for detecting vasospasm in other intracranial arteries are limited, but show a lower sensitivity (13-77%).[50,53-55] ***A negative TCD study does not exclude vasospasm.*** Sources of error are: 1) a tortuous or aberrant artery; 2) distal branch vasospasm; 3) increased intracranial pressure; and 4) a reduction in volume flow (with or without infarction).

Acute Stroke

The intravenous administration of tissue plasminogen activator (tPA) has been shown to dissolve thrombi and improve the long-term outcome of patients with acute ischemic stroke.[56] This can be attributed to early brain tissue reperfusion and arterial recanalization.[56-58] Transcranial Doppler has been used to continuously monitor recanalization during thrombolysis,[59-63] and has a reported sensitivity of 91% and a specificity of 93% in determining complete recanalization of the MCA in patients receiving treatment with tPA.[59]

A fast baseline standard TCD examination is performed in the emergency room. Because the examination is being performed bedside in a noisy environment, it is recommended that the operator position himself or herself properly and use headphones to block out extraneous noise. The occlusion is identified and located by the lack of a Doppler signal and residual blood flow is determined by the presence of an abnormal blood flow Doppler signal (blunted, minimal, etc.) in its vicinity. After locating the site of an occlusion, the TCD transducer is fixed in a monitoring head frame. During monitoring, if the patient is restless, the transducer position is readjusted when necessary. TCD monitoring should be recorded using a monitoring software program or by recording the TCD information on videotape.

TCD monitoring is performed at a variable sample volume depth depending on the location of the occlusion (Figure 6-7). If there is a distal M1-M2 occlusion or a occlusion, residual blood flow signals should be located and monitored at 40 to 45 mm. If the proximal M1 segment is occluded, monitoring is performed at 55 to 60 mm. If no MCA Doppler signal is located, monitoring occurs at a depth that is closest to a normal Doppler signal (usually an ACA signal). Depth settings for the basilar artery are 80mm (proximal) or 100 mm (distal).

TCD monitoring is performed during the entire tPA infusion under direct visual control of a sonographer or a treating physician. If the Doppler signal changes, these changes are noted and the time documented. Changes documented should include the new appearance of a signal, an improvement of blood flow velocity, an increase in the intensity of the signal, any change in the waveform shape, and the appearance of embolic signals.

Continuous TCD monitoring provides a unique noninvasive tool to measure the timing and the amount of intracranial arterial recanalization that often leads to early recovery as well as persisting arterial occlusion that bears grim prognosis. In addition, preliminary results

demonstrate that continuous monitoring with TCD may augment the tPA-induced clot lysis

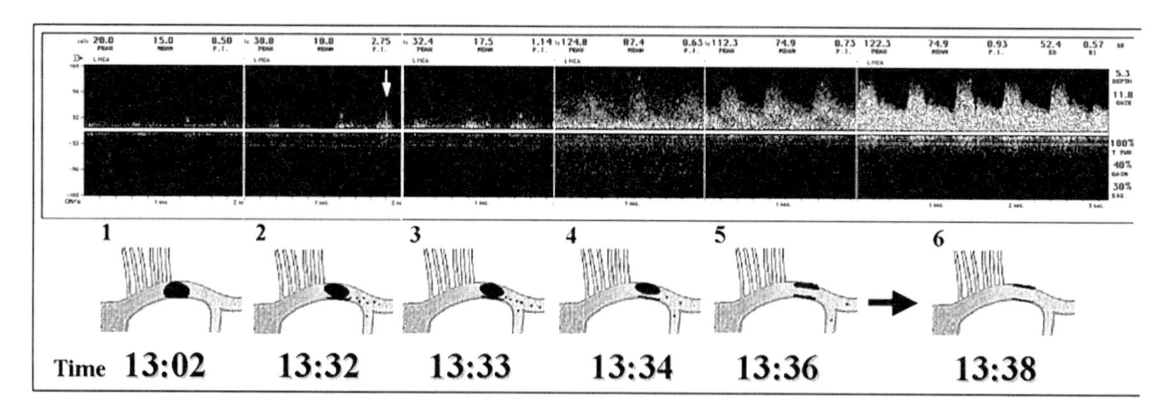

Figure 6-7. The TCD recordings were obtained from the middle cerebral artery (MCA) at a depth of 53 mm from the transtemporal approach. The sample volume size was 11.8mm.

⇒ **Frame 1: Minimal Doppler signal obtained in the proximal MCA at the time of intravenous rtPA bolus.**

⇒ **Frame 2-3: Early restoration of Doppler signals with increasing velocities and microembolic signals (arrow).**

⇒ **Frame 4: MCA Doppler signal continues to improve. There are audible chirping signals (emboli) suggesting continuing clot dissolution.**

⇒ **Frame 5: MCA Doppler signal demonstrates an increased mean velocity above age-expected values and slightly decreased pulsatility indicating distal vasodilation**

⇒ **Frame 6: MCA Doppler signal remains elevated at this time and slightly higher pulsatility suggesting proximal MCA reperfusion with distal vasomotor response.**

since the rates of recanalization and recovery have been shown to be greater than the rates reported when using tPA alone.[61] If this holds true in prospective studies that are now being performed, this opens a new arena for the use of TCD.

Monitoring Changes Of Intracranial Blood Flow/Emboli Detection

The advantage of using TCD as a monitoring tool is that it detects real-time alterations in the cerebral blood supply. Potentially, this information would allow modification of therapy that would benefit the patient. TCD monitoring has been used during carotid endarterectomy, cardiopulmonary bypass, neurosurgical procedures, interventional neuroradiology, and in the intensive care units.

There are several technical points to be made when using TCD during intraoperative monitoring. Patients should have a complete preoperative baseline TCD evaluation. This will give the operator an opportunity to: 1) document the presence of a transtemporal window, 2) become familiar with the patient's intracranial arterial anatomy, 3) obtain baseline velocity values, and 4) evaluate the potential collateral blood flow patterns. Prior to the operative procedure, the location of the transtemporal window should be marked on the patient's skin, which assists in locating the window in the operating room.

On the day of the operation, the TCD operator should be in the operating room early, allowing time to position and set up the equipment. The monitoring performed during operative procedures should be recorded on videotape or by computer tracking. Headphones are used to block out extraneous noise, but often the Doppler signal is audible in the operating room throughout the procedure. If possible, the operator should use a microphone to verbally indicate on the videotape or mark on the computer monitoring, the time when significant operative events occur. It is important that the TCD operator maintains good communication with the surgeon during the operation, so that maneuvers, which might influence intracranial velocities, can be anticipated and accurately recorded.

Modified transducers can be mounted in a headpiece (band, helmet) and placed around the patient's head for continuous MCA monitoring.[64] The operator will need a few minutes to properly position the probe on the patient's head so the middle cerebral artery Doppler signal can be located. A generous amount of ultrasound gel should be applied. Small adjustments of the probe may be necessary during the operative procedure due to inadvertent movement of the patient's head or the headpiece.

The TCD operator must be prepared to hold the probe in place if the headpiece slips during the operation, or if the headpiece interferes with electrode placement for concurrent EEG monitoring. The operator may find that the freehand technique is tiresome if performed during the entire operation. It is, therefore, essential for the TCD operator to be in a comfortable position. We have found the best position is for the operator to sit on a stool at the head of the operating table, stabilizing the examining arm near the patient's head, and using a remote control to operate the TCD equipment. Maintaining a good MCA signal can often be difficult because the surgeon's assistant is often retracting, and her/his hand is directly over the transducer's position. Obviously, the TCD operator's position should not interfere with the anesthesiologist. We therefore recommend the use of small monitoring transducers fixed by durable and tight fixation devices such as Marc series frames by Spencer Technologies. This type of head frame can be adjusted to all commercially available TCD transducers.

Continuous TCD intraoperative monitoring can be technically difficult because of the inability of maintaining constant transducer position for the length of the operation, and electrical interference encountered in the operating room (i.e. electrocautery). Therefore, the most experienced technologist available should be the one involved with intraoperative monitoring.

Intraoperative Monitoring During Carotid Endarterectomy

Most intraoperative TCD monitoring has occurred during carotid endarterectomy.[9,65-82] Middle cerebral artery velocity during cross-clamping might identify patients at risk of suffering an intraoperative stroke due to decreased perfusion, and, therefore, signal the need for carotid shunting.

After locating the best transtemporal window, the MCA velocity is monitored at a depth of 45-55 mm. The Doppler sample volume should not include the terminal-ICA or the ACA. An ischemic index is calculated by expressing the velocity at clamping as a percent of the pre-clamp velocity. The index of ischemia is usually categorized as severe 0-15%, mild 16-40%, and absent if > 40%.

TCD monitoring during carotid endarterectomy has shown that: 1) changes in MCA blood flow velocity can be detected, 2) the MCA velocity change is variable with carotid cross-clamping,[69] 3) MCA velocity changes have had variable correlation with stump pressures, EEG, regional cerebral blood flow, and somatosensory evoked potential (SEP),[66,68,72-76] 4) using better headpieces to hold the transducer in place is critical,[73-76,83] and 5) new insights are being learned regarding the effect of carotid endarterectomy on intracranial hemodynamics.

Detecting the occurrence of microemboli during carotid endarterectomy also has been reported.[65,81,82,84-90] Embolic material has a different acoustic impedance compared to the surrounding blood, causing an identifiable difference in the intensity of the returning Doppler signal.[90] Emboli appear as high-intensity transient signals (HITS) (microembolic signals [MES]) within the Doppler spectral waveform. The Doppler gain should be carefully adjusted to allow visualization of the MES. Emboli may occur at any time during the cardiac cycle and are brief in duration. Emboli sound like a "pop", a "chirp", or a "click" in the audio Doppler signal. Artifacts due to motion, electric interference, and so forth can be differentiated from emboli because the artifacts are usually bi-directional and are predominantly low frequency. During intraoperative monitoring, it should be recorded at what point during the operation the emboli occurred.

Padayachee and colleagues noted air-emboli during shunt insertion in 17 of 19 patients when using TCD monitoring during carotid endarterectomy.[65] In this study, observation of the air emboli signals did not correlate with any adverse postoperative neurologic symptoms in the patients.

Spencer and colleagues reviewed the TCD monitoring videotapes of carotid endarterectomies in 91 patients.[84] Air bubble emboli were found in 56 (62%) patients following the release of cross-clamping. Bubble emboli have high amplitudes and were associated with invasion of the artery wall (release of cross-clamps after arteriotomy closure, insertion of the shunt, etc.). Cerebrovascular symptoms were present postoperatively in one patient who had bubble embolic signals. Additionally, the authors observed formed-element emboli in 24 (26%) patients. Formed-element signals have lower amplitudes and occurred before invasion of the artery wall or several hours after arteriotomy closure. Eleven of these patients had the formed-element signal appear prior to the arteriotomy, and the signals disappeared when manipulation of the artery stopped. Formed-element emboli were observed during extended postoperative periods in two patients, both of who sustained severe strokes. This retrospective study demonstrates that air bubble emboli do not necessarily produce postoperative symptoms, and that patients with persistent postoperative formed-element emboli may be at risk for postoperative cerebrovasular symptoms.

Gaunt and colleagues monitored 91 patients undergoing carotid endarterectomy.[86] Twenty-three patients had particulate emboli during the carotid dissection, which correlated with a significant deterioration in postoperative cognitive function in 11 of the 23 patients. Jansen and colleagues monitored 98 patients undergoing carotid endarterectomy.[85] In this study, all patients had preoperative and postoperative brain imaging. More than ten embolic signals observed during the dissection phase of the operation correlated with new ischemic lesions postoperatively.

Ackerstaff and colleagues performed a prospective study of MCA monitoring during 301 carotid endarterectomies.[87] During this study, more than ten microemboli during the dissection phase were associated with both intraoperative ($p<0.002$) and postoperative ($p<0.02$) cerebral complications. Additionally, greater than 10 microemboli during the dissection phase was significantly ($p<0.005$) related to new hyperintense lesions on postoperative T2-weighted magnetic resonance images. These investigators also found that microemboli occurring during shunting were significantly ($p<0.007$) related to intraoperative complications.

How detecting cerebral emboli influences patient management remains to be determined. The challenge is to use this information to modify surgical technique in order to reduce the risk of stroke in patients undergoing carotid endarterectomy. Ackerstaff and colleagues modified their surgical technique by listening to the audible TCD signal in the operating room during carotid endarterectomies and reduced the intraoperative stroke rate from 4.8% to 1% in their study.[87]

Transcranial Doppler also has been used following carotid endarterectomy to monitor patients with suspected cerebral hyperperfusion.[91-93] This complication results from restored normal cerebral perfusion into a chronically vasodilated tissue bed following carotid endarterectomy. The clinical syndrome may include unilateral headache or face pain, seizures, and delayed cerebral hemorrhage. Although cerebral hyperperfusion following carotid endarterectomy does not occur often, it can lead to serious neurologic complications. The MCA velocities in these patients are significantly increased from preoperative values, and monitoring the MCA velocities can be used to guide therapy.

Monitoring During Cardiopulmonary Bypass

TCD monitoring during cardiac procedures has been limited. Intraoperative monitoring has been used to investigate intracranial hemodynamics to lead to a better understanding of the pathophysiology of the neurologic complications that occur with cardiopulmonary bypass.[94-105] The MCA velocity is monitored for changes in velocity and for emboli identification.

To evaluate the effects of extracranial carotid stenosis during cardiopulmonary bypass, von Reutern and colleagues monitored MCA velocities in 42 patients with less than 50% carotid stenosis, and in 16 patients with a severe stenosis or occlusion of the ICA.[96] Reduced perfusion due to carotid obstruction was not observed during the cardiac procedure suggesting that, in these patients, the carotid disease was not a risk factor for an intra-operative stroke.

Microemboli have been detected during cardiopulmonary bypass surgery. Emboli have been recorded during cannulation of the aorta, at the initiation of bypass, during bypass, at the removal of aortic cross-clamps, and during redistribution of blood from the heart-lung machine to the patient when the heart begins to contract.[97-104]

Pugsley and colleagues monitored the MCA in 105 patients undergoing elective coronary artery surgery.[101] The patients were randomized into two groups. The first group had a 40 micron screen filter placed in the arterial line of the cardiopulmonary bypass circuit, and no filter was used in the second group. A neurologic examination was performed preoperatively, on the first and eighth postoperative day, and at eight weeks after surgery. Patients without the arterial line filter had significantly more neuropsychological deficits at 8 days ($p<0.05$), and at 8 weeks ($p<0.03$), than did the patients with the filter. Additionally, an increase in the number of MES during the cardiopulmonary bypass was related to the likelihood of a patient having a neuropsychological deficit at 8 weeks.

Monitoring During Neurosurgical Procedures

Although monitoring with TCD during neurosurgical, and in association with interventional neuroradiologic procedures is new and investigative, it may provide useful information regarding procedure events that affect cerebral blood flow, and might increase our understanding of cerebral physiology.[105-112]

Giller evaluated the contralateral MCA velocity during 12 craniotomies.[105] The author observed that MCA velocities varied in accordance with known CBF changes from a variety of intraoperative events, and that TCD provided insight regarding cerebral autoregulation.

Surgical sacrifice of the carotid artery is often anticipated during treatment of complex tumors and aneurysms. Currently, trial occlusion of the carotid artery with a balloon during arteriography is performed with concurrent neurologic examination or cerebral blood flow measurement. TCD changes during trial carotid occlusion could allow patients to be stratified according to their risk, and thereby might predict the clinical response to carotid artery occlusion. Giller and colleagues monitored MCA velocities during manual common carotid compression of 22 patients and compared it to balloon occlusion of the cervical ICA.[106] The balloon occlusion was continued for 30-45 minutes or until a focal deficit was observed. SPECT studies were obtained at baseline and during balloon occlusion in 14 patients. Less than a 65% reduction in MCA velocity was obtained in fifteen patients, and 93% (14/15) of these patients tolerated the balloon occlusion without clinical deterioration. Seven patients had a ≥65% reduction of MCA velocity, and 86% (6/7) developed a transient focal deficit during balloon occlusion. This study suggests that a decrease of more than 65% of the MCA velocity during transient manual compression of the CCA correlates with a significant impairment of perfusion.

Emboli Detection

Emboli detection has been reported during routine TCD testing in patients with carotid and cardiac disease.[113-138] When monitoring the MCA for emboli, it is best to use the main trunk of the MCA (45-55mm). A headband or helmet is recommended to hold the transducer in place since a minimum of 15 to 20 minutes of monitoring is required. Videotape recording or computer tracking is essential and the emboli rate is reported as the number of emboli per hour. Monitoring software that automatically counts the number of MES is available for many TCD instruments. Remember, emboli cause an identifiable difference in the intensity of the returning Doppler signal. Therefore, proper Doppler gain setting is critical and should be reduced so that the emboli can be detected.

The Consensus Committee of the Ninth International Cerebral Hemodynamic Symposium proposed minimal identification criteria for establishing microembolic signals (Figure 6-8).[140] An individual Doppler microembolic signal must have the following four features: 1) the signal is transient, usually lasting less than 300 microseconds, 2) the amplitude of the signal is at least 3dB higher than the background blood flow signal, 3) the signal is unidirectional within the Doppler spectral waveform; and 4) a microembolic signal is accompanied by a "snap", "chirp", or "moan" on the audio output.

Markus and colleagues monitored bilateral MCAs for 20 minutes on each side.[113] No emboli were detected in 20 normal volunteers. However, emboli were detected in 24% (6/25) of the symptomatic patients with a carotid stenosis (mean=2.17 signals per 20 minutes), and in 38% (9/24) of the patients with prosthetic cardiac valves (mechanical valves; mean=17.6 signals per 20 minutes).

Siebler and colleagues monitored the MCA for one hour in 20 controls, 33 symptomatic patients, and 56 asymptomatic patients.[114] All patients had an extracranial ICA stenosis. There were no emboli detected in the controls. However, emboli were observed in 16% (9/56) of the asymptomatic patients and in 80% (27/33) of the symptomatic patients.

Additionally, Siebler and colleagues followed 64 asymptomatic patients for a mean follow-up of 72 weeks.[115] The patients had a documented unilateral 70-99% stenosis of the extracranial ICA by carotid duplex imaging, and did not have a history of atrial fibrillation or an artificial heart valve. The MCA was monitored for one hour. Thirteen percent (8/64) had ≥ 2 emboli per hour. This study demonstrated a significant association between ≥ 2 emboli per

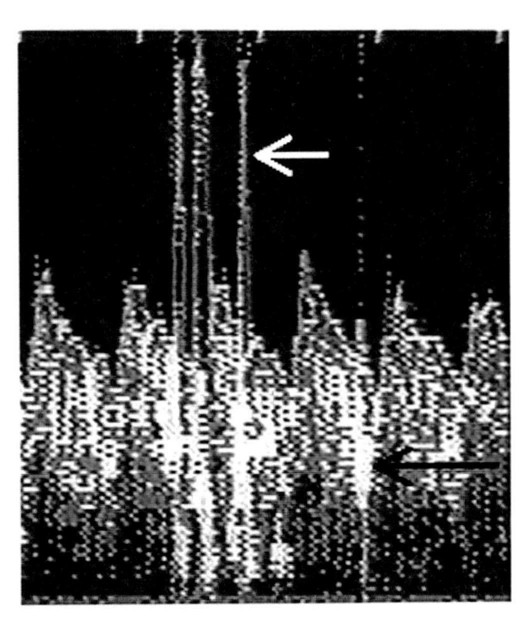

Figure 6-8. Emboli signals (black arrow) within a MCA Doppler spectral waveform. The Doppler gain setting was too high producing artifacts (white arrow).

hour detected during a TCD examination and a subsequent neurologic event (p=0.005).

Valton and colleagues monitored 48 MCAs in 26 asymptomatic and symptomatic patients who underwent selective carotid arteriography.[116] Embolic signals were detected in 8 MCAs. An ulcerated plaque was found on arteriography in 5 out of 8 (63%) cases with embolic signals and in 9 out of 40 (23%) without embolic signals (p=0.02).

Sitzer and colleagues monitored the MCA ipsilateral to a high grade extracranial ICA stenosis.[117] In this study of asymptomatic and symptomatic patients, the investigators compared the relationship between preoperative microembolic rates per hour (0, ≤ 5, >5) and the pathoanatomic features of 38 carotid artery endarterectomy specimens. There was a significant (p ≤ 0.005) association between cerebral microemboli and ulceration and intraluminal thrombus found in the specimen. There was no significant correlation between microemboli and plaque fissure or intraplaque hemorrhage.

Forteza and colleagues reviewed 69 arteries in 66 symptomatic patients.[128] All patients had undergone TCD monitoring for thirty minutes as part of their neurological evaluation. HITS were identified in 20 of 69 (29%) of the arteries. The median interval between onset of symptoms and time of TCD testing was 4 days (range 0.16 to 45 days) for HITS-positive arteries, and 12 days (range 1 to 1080 days) for HITS-negative arteries. The difference between the two groups was significant (p=0.0046). Additionally, in this study, 14 of 32 (44%) arteries in patients with transient ischemic attacks, and 6 of 37 (16%) arteries in patients with cerebral infarctions, were HITS-positive (p=0.012). These investigators demonstrated that microembolic signals are more frequently detected when patients are evaluated soon after the initiation of symptoms, and that embolic signals are detected more frequently in patients presenting with transient hemispheric or retinal ischemia versus those with cerebral infarction.

The detection of cerebral microemboli by TCD offers new information in the diagnosis and management of patients with cerebrovascular disease. Good inter-observer agreement suggests that the detection of microemboli by TCD is sufficiently reproducible to be used in the clinical setting.[141,142] Additional prospective studies are needed to define the risk of MES as a factor for stroke. Adding the potential advantage of microemboli detection to TCD monitoring must be balanced with known limitations.[143-145]

Subclavian Steal

The subclavian steal syndrome is characterized by symptoms of brain stem ischemia associated with a stenosis or occlusion of the left subclavian, the innominate, or the right subclavian arteries proximal to the origin of the vertebral artery. A stenosis at this location may cause the pressure in the upper extremity to be lower than normal. The production of this pressure gradient can cause reversal of flow in the vertebral artery especially during exercise of the involved arm. If this occurs, the vertebral artery becomes a major collateral to the upper extremity. The "stealing" of blood from the basilar artery, via retrograde vertebral artery flow, causes the patient to experience neurological symptoms of brain stem ischemia.

Upper extremity pulses are palpated, and bilateral blood pressures are recorded. The most constant physical finding of subclavian steal is a difference in arm systolic pressures of ≥ 20 mmHg. If a systolic pressure differential of ≥ 20 mmHg between brachial arteries is detected, a subclavian or innominate artery obstruction on the side with the lower pressure should be suspected. This physical finding is absent in rare instances and in cases of bilateral lesions.

If subclavian steal is suspected, a standard TCD examination should be performed with special attention focused on the blood flow direction and velocities in the vertebral and the basilar arteries. Blood flow is normally away from the transducer (suboccipital approach) in the vertebrobasilar system. If blood flow is toward the transducer in a vertebral or basilar artery, then there is evidence of a steal. Often the reversed blood flow direction is found only in a vertebral artery, suggesting a possible vertebral to vertebral steal.

In the absence of flow reversal at rest, or if alternating blood flow direction is observed, the involved upper extremity should be stressed to reduce outflow resistance, thereby revealing the hemodynamics of a potentially latent steal. The baseline examination and the subsequent changes in the spectral waveforms, which occur following arm exercise or post-occlusive hyperemia, are recorded on videotape or by computer tracking. Post-occlusive reactive hyperemia is preferred in this setting. A blood pressure cuff is applied to the arm ipsilateral to the arterial stenosis/occlusion. The ipsilateral vertebral Doppler signal is located and monitored during inflation of the arm cuff. The blood pressure cuff is inflated above systolic pressure (>20 mmHg above systolic) for approximately three minutes, and any changes in the Doppler signal are noted. Then the cuff is rapidly deflated (quickly released from the arm) and changes in vertebral artery blood flow direction and velocity are recorded. This procedure is repeated with monitoring of the contralateral vertebral artery and the basilar artery. A 5-10 minute rest period between evaluations is necessary for the return of baseline arterial hemodynamics between evaluations.

The role of basilar artery blood flow in suspected subclavian steal can be documented by transcranial Doppler.[9,146-150] Resting basilar artery blood flow is rarely affected, but may become abnormal after reactive hyperemia testing if the contralateral feeding vertebral artery is also diseased. Reports have demonstrated that basilar artery blood flow is resistant to velocity changes due to subclavian steal, and that reversal of basilar artery blood flow is rare.[9,146]

Ringelstein and colleagues demonstrated a subclavian steal by TCD in 91 patients.[9] Alternating blood flow or complete reversal of blood flow direction in the basilar artery was demonstrated in only one of 48 cases of latent steal (transient decelerated or reversed flow in the stealing vertebral artery). Blood flow direction in the basilar was alternating or completely reversed in 12 of the remaining 43 patients with a steal (permanently reversed flow in the stealing vertebral artery). Additionally, these 12 patients had disease of the contralateral subclavian or feeding vertebral artery. In this study, alternating or reversal of blood flow in the basilar artery was not a common finding in patients with a documented steal, unless there was hemodynamically significant disease of the feeding vertebral artery or the contralateral subclavian artery.

In most patients, subclavian steal appears to be a harmless hemodynamic phenomenon. However, its proper documentation shows a widespread atherosclerotic process that may affect major aortic branches and have implications for patient management. If symptomatic subclavian steal can be corrected by balloon angioplasty or stenting of the subclavian artery.

Arteriovenous Malformations

An arteriovenous malformation (AVM) is a developmental anomaly (collection of abnormal vessels) in which blood flows directly from the arterial circulation to the venous circulation without intervening capillaries. In an AVM, the resistance is low compared with normal cerebrovascular resistance. Arteries that supply the AVM are termed "feeders" to distinguish them from the arteries supplying the surrounding neural tissue. Because they carry a large volume of blood flow, feeders are large diameter arteries and are characterized by an increased velocity, reduced pulsatility, and reduced responsiveness to CO_2.[151-156] The venous drainage is comprised of enlarged veins that carry pulsatile arterialized blood. The danger is that the tissue normally supplied by the involved arterial circulation may become ischemic if the shunt produced by the AVM is severe.

TCD demonstrates the hemodynamics of the AVM, as well as its anatomic location. A standard TCD examination is performed in these patients with attention given to the intracranial arterial velocities, pulsatility indices, and direction of flow. Increased velocities often approach the magnitude like those associated with vasospasm following subarachnoid hemorrhage, but the P.I. tends to be lower since vascular resistance is low.

Pioneering transcranial Doppler studies enthusiastically endorsed a potential role for TCD to detect AVM's, the promise that did not hold true. The sensitivity of detecting intracranial AVMs relies on the ability of TCD to detect it feeder. Its detection depends on AVM size, location, and the number and length of the main feeders. Lindegaard and colleagues reported that TCD detected 93% (26/28) of the AVMs evaluated.[151] In their study, both the AVMs not detected were less than 2 cm.

Petty and colleagues studied 15 patients (19 feeding arteries) with AVMs and evaluated the outcome of therapy, comparing the final hemodynamics of those treated with embolization (10 feeding arteries) compared to surgical resection (9 feeding arteries).[152] The initial diagnosis and treatment outcome were confirmed arteriographically in all patients. Post-treatment TCD examinations were performed on average eight days following treatment. Both surgery and embolization resulted in similar changes in hemodynamics, demonstrating a decrease in velocity and an increase in the pulsatility indices. Although there were greater hemodynamic changes in the surgically treated group, this trend did not reach statistical significance. The authors of this study demonstrated that TCD, as compared to arteriography, could reliably evaluate the hemodynamic outcome of treatment of AVMs.

Mast and colleagues prospectively evaluated 114 consecutive AVM patients, 22 non-AVM patients with acute cerebral hemorrhage, and 52 normal subjects.[155] The sensitivity for detecting large (>5cm) and medium-sized (2.6 to 5 cm) AVMs by TCD was greater than 80%. However, the detection of small (≤ 2.5 cm) AVMs was poor. Additionally, the results of this study support that, in acute cerebral hemorrhage,

TCD may be useful in the differentiation of AVM from non-AVM bleeds, and the study results raise doubts about the concept of a hemodynamic steal in AVMs.

Predicting Stroke in Sickle Cell Disease

TCD and TCDI are being used in the evaluation of children with sickle cell disease.[157-168] Hemoglobin S tends to form intracellular polymers that distort red blood cells, and sickle cell disease is characterized by chronic hemolytic anemia. Cerebral infarction in these patients is associated with an occlusion vasculopathy involving the terminal the middle cerebral artery, and the anterior cerebral arteries. Prevention of stroke may be feasible with transfusion therapy if patients at risk can be identified.

Adams and colleagues performed TCD examinations in 190 patients (age at entry was 3-18 years old) with sickle cell disease.[157] In this study, a TCD examination was considered abnormal if velocities exceeded 170 cm/sec. The TCD was within normal limits in 167 patients and abnormal in 23 patients. The clinical and hematologic considerations were similar between the two groups. In six out of seven of the patients who had a stroke, the TCD was abnormal. The results of this study were helpful in planning a large multi-centered trial of TCD in children with sickle cell disease.

In the **STrOke P**revention trial in sickle cell disease (STOP), Adams and colleagues enrolled 130 children (age 2 to 16) who were found to be a high risk for stroke on the basis of elevated (>200 cm/sec) intracranial arterial mean velocities of the MCA or the .[164] The TCD study had to be positive on two separate occasions. The children were randomized to receive either standard supportive care or periodic blood transfusions. After one year, 10 children in the standard care group had a cerebral infarction compared to one child in the transfusion group. A clinical alert was released on September 18, 1997 from the National Heart, Lung and Blood Institute.[167] The clinical alert announced that periodic red blood cell transfusions to maintain the level of hemoglobin S (HbS) below 30%, reduced the rate of cerebral infarction by 90% in children found to be at increased risk by virtue of having elevated intracranial arterial velocities.

It is now recommended that children (ages 2-16) with sickle cell disease (SS or Sß°) undergo annual screening with TCD. If the TCD examination is positive, ≥ 200cm/s in the MCA or on two separate occasions, the child is at high risk for developing a stroke (Figure 6-9). The decision to begin a child on chronic blood transfusion therapy is a clinical decision that should be made after careful consideration of the risks and benefits. When performing TCD examinations in children, several changes in technique that will improve the quality of the examination. Before beginning the TCD examination, the test should be explained to the child and the caregiver. To reduce fear and anxiety, allowing the child to touch the gel, listen to the Doppler signals, and observe the transducer being used on someone else.

Prior to beginning the examination it is necessary to measure the child's head. As children grow and their heads become larger, the bitemporal measurement is necessary to define the depth of the patient's midline (half the bitemporal measurement). This measurement is critical to accurately perform a TCD examination in a child, because with large transtemporal windows, it easy to move

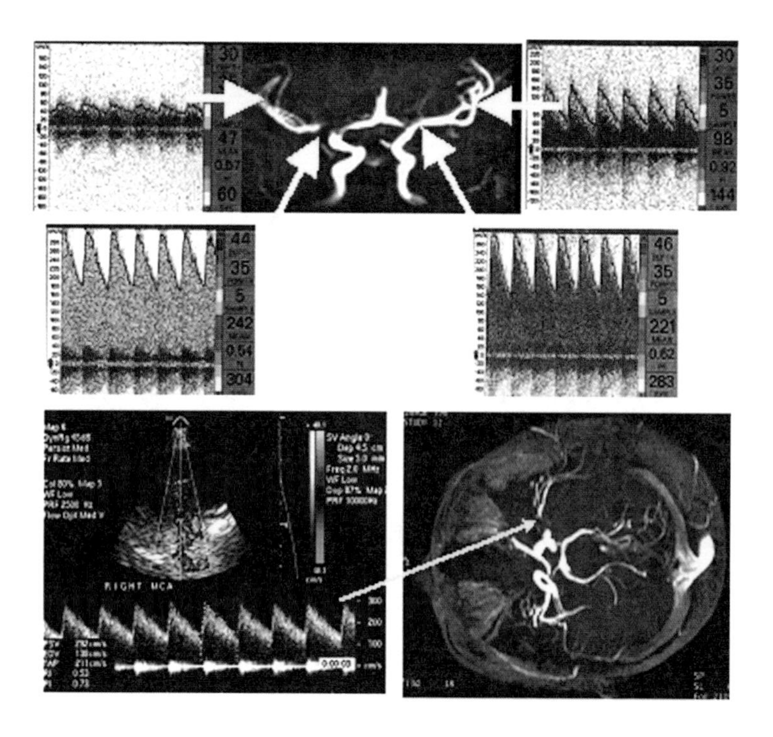

Figure 6-9. TCD and TCDI identified intracranial arterial narrowings in a child with sickle cell disease. Mean velocity in the middle cerebral artery was greater than 200 cm/sec bilaterally.

across midline and evaluate the contralateral arteries by error. In addition, the expected depth range for the intracranial arteries will vary as the child's head diameter increases.

The TCD windows are usually large and easy to locate in most children. Because of the large windows, the TCD power/ intensity control setting should be reduced. The power/intensity level should be set at a maximum, however, if it is difficult to locate the transtemporal window. Additionally, many children will not tolerate the ultrasound evaluation via the transorbital window. If using this window is necessary in a child, this approach should be used last. When using the transorbital window, the operator is reminded to decrease the Doppler output/intensity level to a minimum.

A technical challenge when performing TCD examinations in children is that often they will only lie still for short time. In some cases, allowing the child to move between the evaluation of the different windows may be beneficial and will improve the quality of the examination. If a child will not lie still or is afraid, the examination may be performed with the child sitting in their caregiver's lap. Although this patient position is not ideal, it is possible to complete the examination with the child in this position. The operator must pay special attention to maintaining proper transducer-to-artery angle when performing the test when the child is in this position.

Additionally, when performing TCD in children, a smaller sample volume size (6 mm) will usually provide good quality Doppler signals. Using a smaller sample volume size will also be useful when trying to isolate the small intracranial arteries.

The operator should also document if the child is crying or falls asleep during the examination, because this will change the patient's cerebral blood flow, and have an affect on the intracranial arterial velocities recorded. If possible, try to reschedule the examination. If the examination must be performed, wake the sleeping patient, and take the time to calm the patient who is afraid.

Intracranial arterial velocities are increased in children. For example, in a child who is 10 year old, the mean velocity in the middle cerebral artery is approximately 95 cm/s. To accurately measure the increased velocities obtained when examining children, the velocity scale needs to be increased or the zero baseline should be lowered to accurately display the spectral Doppler waveform.

Brain Death

Although clinical criteria for brain death have been established,[168] most institutions request that ancillary studies (electroendcephalography, computerized tomography [CT], radioisotopic scan, arteriography, etc.) be used to confirm the diagnosis. These tests, however, are expensive, often cannot be performed bedside, and can be time-consuming. TCD is a noninvasive, portable, less expensive, quick confirmatory test that is easily repeatable. When using TCD in these patients, it is important to recognize that TCD evaluates intracranial velocities (cerebral circulatory arrest) and does not assess brain tissue. Therefore, its findings are not synonymous with tissue death.

Cerebral perfusion pressure (CPP) is the difference between systemic arterial blood pressure (SAP) and the intracranial pressure (ICP). Cerebral circulatory arrest occurs when the intracranial pressure equals or exceeds the systemic arterial pressure.

During normal conditions, the ICP is less than the systemic arterial blood pressure, and end-diastolic flow velocities are approximately 50% of the systolic peak velocity. Increased ICP (increased peripheral resistance) causes a decrease in the diastolic flow velocity, with the systolic peaks of the spectral waveforms assuming a spiky appearance (increased pulsatility). As the ICP increases and approaches the diastolic SAP, the end-diastolic perfusion is reduced. When ICP is equal to the diastolic SAP, diastolic flow velocity disappears and only systolic peaks are detectable. If the ICP continues to increase (a further drop in CPP), a diastolic flow component of the spectral waveform velocity reappears in the reversed direction. This characteristic TCD waveform is often referred to as the *to-and-fro* waveform. This signal reflects the oscillating movement of the blood column in the large intracranial arteries reflected from the arterioles, indicating no perfusion of the brain parenchyma. When the CPP approaches zero, three different TCD waveforms have been described: the oscillatory, or reverberating signal (*to-and-fro*), a short systolic spike signal, or the absence of a signal that was previously present. Variations of these TCD patterns exist, and progression from one stage to the next does not imply irreversible progression to brain death.

Investigators have emphasized that TCD is a method to confirm the clinical diagnosis and is not used alone to make the diagnosis.[170-177] These reports indicate that Doppler signals should be obtained in several intracranial arteries from different windows since the patient population may have variable amounts of associated intracranial disease. The absence of an intracranial Doppler signal does not establish the diagnosis of brain death since differences exist in the technical skill of the examiners, and because there are differences in the ossification of the temporal bone between patients. The study by Powers and colleagues suggested that representative TCD signals alone were inadequate, and that Doppler signals with a net flow velocity of less than 10 cm/sec in the MCA was found to be sensitive determinant of brain death.[173]

Patients are usually evaluated bedside in the intensive care unit. The operator is reminded to: 1) be properly positioned, 2) correct for transducer-artery angles that may be affected by a change in operator position, 3) use headphones to reduce extraneous noise, 4) use a remote control for ease of operation, 5) mark the patient's skin, indicating the location of the transtemporal window, making it possible to perform accurate, repeatable studies, 6) make recordings from several intracranial arteries using different TCD windows, and 7) repeat examinations to avoid false positive tests.

It is evident that when decisions about life or death are being made, all sources of error must be eliminated. As previously discussed, variability of intracranial anatomy, inadequate transtemporal windows, and inexperienced examiners are common factors leading to inaccurate results. To date, clinicians have not relied upon TCD as the only objective confirmation of their clinical impression, and additional correlations are required. Repeated examinations in patients with severe brain injury will undoubtedly offer insight to their prognoses and the natural history of their injuries.

Summary

Currently, TCD is used for a variety of clinical indications. Despite growth in experience and improvements in technique and equipment, clinical usefulness of TCD remains controversial. Its clinical value is associated with monitoring patients for vasospasm, screening children with sickle cell disease, and the evaluation of patients with intracranial disease. TCD may be useful in the future for confirmation of brain death, monitoring during surgical and radiologic procedures, and in the evaluation of patients with migraine headaches.

It is apparent that TCD is not useful as a routine screening test as part of the noninvasive cerebrovascular evaluation, since the incidence of intracranial disease is low and the older patients present with technical challenges. While the past twenty years has lead to a proliferation of research using TCD, at this time its clinical role still remains questionable concerning how the TCD examination fits into the workup for the spectrum of cerebrovascular disease.

References

1. Kaps M, Damian MS, Teschendorf U, Dorndorf W. Transcranial Doppler ultrasound findings in middle cerebral artery occlusion.Stroke 1990;21:532-537.

2. Lindegaard K-F, Bakke SJ, Aaslid R, Nornes H. Doppler diagnosis of intracranial artery occlusive disorders. J Neurol Neurosurg Psychiatry 1986;49:510-518.

3. Spencer MP, Whisler D. Transorbital Doppler diagnosis of intracranial arterial stenosis. Stroke 1986;17(5): 916-921.

4. Hennerici M, Rautenber W, Schwartz A. Transcranial Doppler ultrasound for the assessment of intracranial arterial flow velocity - Part 2. Evaluation of intracranial arterial disease. Surg Neurol 1987;27:523-532.

5. Grolimund P, Seiler RW, Aaslid R, et al. Evaluation of cerebrovascular disease by combined extracranial and transcranial Doppler sonography. Experience in 1,039 patients. Stroke 1987;18:1018-1024.

6. de Bray J-M, Joseph P-A, Jeanvoine H, et al. Transcranial Doppler evaluation of middle cerebral artery stenosis. J Ultrasound Med 1988;7:611-616.

7. Mattle H, Grolimund P, Huber P, et al. Transcranial Doppler sonographic findings in middle cerebral artery disease. Arch Neurol 1988;45:289-295.

8. Kirkham FJ, Neville BGR, Levin SD. Bedside diagnosis of stenosis of middle cerebral artery. The Lancet (Letter) 1986;797-798.

9. Ringelstein EB. A Practical Guide To Transcranial Doppler Sonography. In: Weinberger J (Ed) Noninvasive Imaging Of Cerebrovascular Disease. A. Liss Publishers, New York, 1989:75-121.

10. Mull M, Aulich A, Hennerici M. Transcranial Doppler ultrasonography versus arteriography for assessment of the vertebrobasilar circulation. J Clin Ultrasound 1990;18:539-549.

11. Ley-Pozo J, Ringelstein EB. Noninvasive detection of occlusive disease of the carotid siphon and middle cerebral artery. Ann Neurol 1990;28:640-647.

12. Rorick MB, Nichols FT, Adams RJ. Transcranial Doppler correlation with angiography in detection of intracranial stenosis. Stroke 1994;25:1931-1934.

13. Baumgartner RW, Mattle HP, Schroth G. Assessment of =50% and <50% intracranial stenoses by transcranial color-coded duplex sonography. Stroke 1999;30:87-92.

14. Arenillas JF, Molina CA, Montaner J, et al. Progression and clinical recurrence of symptomatic middle cerebral artery stenosis: a long-term follow-up transcranial Doppler ultrasound study. Stroke 2001;32:2898-2904.

15. Harders A. Neurosurgical applications of transcranial Doppler sonography. Intra-aneurysmal flow pattern. New York: Springer-Verlag, 1986:72-75.

16. Baumgartner RW, Mattle HP, Kothbauer K, Schroth G. Transcranial color-coded duplex sonography in cerebral aneurysms. Stroke 1994;25:2429-2434.

17. Martin PJ, Gaunt ME, Naylor AR et al. Intracranial aneurysms and arterio-venous malformations: transcranial colour-coded sonography as a diagnostic aid. Ultrasound Med Biol 1994;20:689-698.

18. Becker G, Greiner K, Kuane B, et al. Diagnosis and monitoring of subarachnoid hemorrhage by transcranial color-coded real-time sonography. Neurosurgery 1999;28: 814 -820.

19. Wardlaw JM, Cannon JC. Color transcranial "power" Doppler ultrasound of intracranial aneurysms. J Neurosurg. 1996;84:459-461.

20. Lindegaard K-F, Bakke SJ, Grolimund P, et al. Assessment of intracranial hemodynamics in carotid artery disease by transcranial Doppler ultrasound. J Neurosurg 1985;63:890-898.

21. Babikian V, Sloan MA, Tegeler CH, et al. Transcranial Doppler validation pilot study. J Neuroimag 1993;3:242-249.

22. Reith W, Pfadenhauer K, Loeprecht H. Significance of transcranial Doppler CO_2 reactivity measurements for the diagnosis of hemodynamically relevant carotid obstructions. Ann Vasc Surg 1990;4:359-364.

23. Widder B. The Doppler CO_2 test to exclude patients not in need of extracranial/intracranial bypass surgery. J Neurol, Neurosurg and Psychiatry 1989;52:38-42.

24. Visser GH, van Huffelen AC, Wieneke GH, Eikelboom BC. Bilateral increase in CO_2 reactivity after unilateral carotid endarterectomy. Stroke 1997;28:899-905.

25. White RP, Markus HS. Impaired dynamic cerebral autoregulation in carotid artery stenosis. Stroke 1997;28:1340-1344.

26. Ringelstein EB, Sievers C, Ecker S, et al. Noninvasive assessment of CO_2-induced cerebral vasomotor response in normal individuals and patients with occlusions. Stroke 1988;19:963-969.

27. Vriens EM, Kraaier V, Musbach M, et al. Transcranial pulsed Doppler measurements of blood velocity in the middle cerebral artery: ref. values at rest and during hyperventilation in healthy volunteers in relation to age and sex. Ultrasound Med Biol. 1989; 15(1):1-8.

28. Huber P, Handa J. Effect of contrast material, hypercapnia,hyperventilation, hypertonic glucose and papaverine on the diameter of the cerebral arteries. Angiographic determination in man. Invest Radiol 1967;2:17-32

29. Markwalder T-M, Grolimund P, Seiler RW et al. Dependency of blood flow velocity in the middle cerebral artery on end-tidal carbon dioxide partial pressure-a transcranial ultrasound Doppler study. J Cereb Blood Flow Metab 1984;4:368-372.

30. Markus HS, Harrison MJG. Estimation of cerebrovascular reactivity using transcranial Doppler, including the use of breath-holding as the vasodilatory stimulus. Stroke 1992;23:668-673.

31. Bishop CCR, Powell S, Insall M, et al. Effect of occlusion on middle cerebral artery blood flow at rest and in response to hypercapnia. Lancet 1986;710-712.

32. Silvestrini M, Vernieri F, Pasqualetti P, et al. Impaired cerebral vasoreactivity and risk of stroke in patients with asymptomatic carotid artery stenosis. JAMA 2000; 283:2122-2127.

33. Vernieri F, Pasqualetti P, Matteis M, et al. Effect of collateral blood flow and cerebral vasomotor reactivity on the outcome of carotid artery occlusion. Stroke 2001;32:1552-1558.

34. Kleisser B, Widder B. Course of carotid artery occlusions with impaired cerebrovascular reactivity. Stroke 1992;23:171-174.

35. Eskesin V et al. Observer variability in assessment of angiographic vasospasm after aneurysmal subarachnoid haemorrhage. Acta Neurochir 1987; 87:54-57.

36. Aaslid R, Huber P, Nornes H. Evaluation of cerebrovascular vasospasm with transcranial Doppler ultrasound. J Neurosurg 1984;60:37-41.

37. Aaslid R, Huber P, Nornes H. A transcranial Doppler method in the evaluation of cerebrovascular vasospasm. Neuroradiology 1986;28: 11-16.

38. Seiler RW, Grolimund P, Aaslid R, Huber P, Nornes H. Cerebral vasospasm evaluated by transcranial ultrasound correlated with clinical grade and CT-visualized subarachnoid hemorrhage. J Neurosurg 1986;64:594-600.

39. Harders AG, Gilsbach JM. Time course of blood velocity changes related to vasospasm in the circle of Willis measured by transcranial Doppler ultrasound. J Neurosurg 1987; 66:718-728.

40. Sekhar LN, Wechsler LR, Yonas H, et al. Value of transcranial Doppler examination in the diagnosis of cerebral vasospasm after subarachnoid hemorrhage. Neurosurg 1988;22:813-821.

41. Romner B, Ljunggren B, Brandt L, Saveland H. Transcranial Doppler sonography within 12 hours after subarachnoid hemorrhage. J Neurosurg 1989;70:732-736.

42. Sloan MA, Haley EC, Kassell NF, et al. Sensitivity and specificity of transcranial Doppler ultrasonography in the diagnosis of vasospasm following subarachnoid hemorrhage. Neurology 1989;39:1514-1518.

43. Newell DW, Winn HR. Transcranial Doppler in cerebral vasospasm. Neurosurgery Clinics of North America 1990;1(2):319-328.

44. Seiler RW, Nirkko AC. Effect of Nimodipine on cerebrovascular response to CO_2 in asymptomatic individuals and patients with subarachnoid hemorrhage: A transcranial Doppler ultrasound study. Neurosurg 1990;27:247-251.

45. Aaslid R, Nornes H. Musical murmurs in human cerebral arteries after subarachnoid hemorrhage. J Neurosurg 1984;60:32-36.

46. Creissard P, Proust F. Vasospasm diagnosis: theoretical sensitivity of transcranial Doppler evaluated using 135 angiograms demonstrating vasospasm. Acta Neurochir 1994; 131:12-18.

47. Ekelund A, Saveland H, Romner B, Brandt L. Transcranial Doppler ultrasound in hypertensive versus normotensive patients after aneurysmal subarachnoid hemorrhage. Stroke 1995;26:2071-2074.

48. Lindegaard KF, Nornes H, Bakke SJ, et al. Cerebral vasospasm diagnosis by means of angiography and blood velocity measurements. Acta Neurochir 1989;100:12-24.

49. Sloan MA, Zagardo MT, Wozniak MA, et al. Sensitivity and specificity of flow velocity ratios for the diagnosis of vasospasm after subarachnoid hemorrhage: preliminary report. In: Klingelhofer J, Bartles E, Ringelstein EB (Eds). New Trends in Cerebral Hemodynamics and Neurosonology. Amsterdam: Elsevier. 1997;221-227.

50. Soustiel JF, Shik V, Shreiber R, Tavor Y. Basilar vasospasm diagnosis: investigation of a modified "Lindegaard Index" based on imaging studies and blood velocity measurements of the basilar artery. Stroke. 2002;33:72-7.

51. Burch CM, Wozniak MA, Sloan MA et al. Detection of intracranial and middle cerebral artery vasospasm following subarachnoid hemorrhage. J Neuro imaging 1996;6:8-15.

52. Compton JS, Redmond S, Symon L. Cerebral blood velocity in subarachnoid haemorrhage: a transcranial Doppler study. J Neurol Neurosurg Psychiatry 1987;50:1499-1503.

53. Lennihan L, Petty GW, Fink ME et al. Transcranial Doppler detection of anterior cerebral artery vasospasm. J Neurol Neurosurg Psychiatry 1993; 56:906-909.

54. Sloan MA, Burch CH, Wozniak MA, et al. Transcranial Doppler detection of vertebrobasilar vasospasm following subarachnoid hemorrhage. Stroke 1994;25:2187-2197.

55. Muizelaar J. The need for a quantifiable normalized transcranial Doppler ratio for the diagnosis of posterior circulation vasospasm. Stroke 2002;33:78.

56. The National Institute of Neurological Disorders and Stroke re-PA Stroke Study Group. Tissue plasminogen activator for acute ischemic stroke. N Engl J Med 1995;333:1581-1587.

57. Grotta JC, Alexandrov AV. TPA-associated reperfusion in acute ischemic stroke demonstrated by SPECT. Stroke 1998;29:429-432.

58. Demchuk AM, Felberg RA, Alexandrov AV. Clinical recovery from acute ischemic stroke after early reperfusion of the brain with intravenous thrombolysis. N Engl J Med. 1999;340:894-895.

59. Burgin SW, Felberg RA, Demchuk A, et al. Ultrasound criteria for middle cerebral artery recanalization: an angiographic correlation. Stroke 2000;31:329.

60. Cintas P, Le Traon AP, Larrue V. High rate of recanalization of middle cerebral artery occlusion during 2-MHz transcranial color-coded Doppler continuous monitoring without thrombolytic drug. Stroke 2002;33: 626-628.

61. Alexandrov AV, Demchuk AM, Felber RA, et al. High rate of complete recanalization and dramatic clinical recovery during tPA infusion when continuously monitored with 2-MHz transcranial Doppler monitoring. Stroke 2000;31:610-61.

62. Alexandrov AV, Burgin WS, Demchuk AM, et al. Speed of intracranial clot lysis with intravenous tissue plasminogen activator therapy. Sonographic classification and short-term improvement. Circulation 2001; 103:2897-2902.

63. El-Mitwalli A, Saad M, Christou I, et al. Clinical and sonographic patterns of tandem /middle cerebral artery occlusion in tissue plasminogen activator-treated patients. Stroke 2002;33:99-102.

64. Giller CA, Giller AM. A new method for fixation of probes for transcranial Doppler ultrasound. J Neuroimaging 1997;7:103-105.

65. Padayachee TS, Gosling RG, Bishop CC, et al. Monitoring middle cerebral artery blood velocity during carotid endarterectomy. Br J Surg 1986;73:98-100.

66. Padayachee TS, Gosling RG, Lewis RR, et al. Transcranial Doppler assessment of cerebral collateral during carotid endarterectomy. Br J Surg 1987;74:260-262.

67. Bass A, Krupski WC, Schneider PA, et al. Intraoperative transcranial Doppler: Limitations of the method. J Vasc Surg 1989;10:549-553.

68. Halsey JH, McDowell HA, Gelmon S, Morawetz RB. Blood velocity in the middle cerebral artery and regional blood flow during carotid endarterectomy. Stroke 1989;20:53-58.

69. deBorst GJ, Moll FL, van de Pavoordt HD, et al. Stroke from carotid endarterectomy: when and how to reduce perioperative stroke rate? Eur J Vasc Endovasc Surg 2001;21:484-489.

70. Ringelstein EB. Transcranial Doppler Monitoring. Chapter 10. In: Aaslid R (Ed), Transcranial Doppler Sonography New York:Springer Verlag, 1986:147-163.

71. Schneider PA, Rossman ME, Torem S, et al. Transcranial Doppler in the management of extracranial cerebrovascular disease: implications in diagnosis and monitoring. J Vasc Surg 1988;7:223-231.

72. Thiel A, Russ W, Zeiler D, et al. Transcranial Doppler sonography and somatosensory evoked potential monitoring in carotid surgery. Eur J Vasc Surg 1990;4:597-602.

73. Schneider PA, Ringelstein EB, Rossman ME, et al. Importance of cerebral collateral pathways during carotid endarterectomy. Stroke 1988;19:1328-1334.

74. Jansen C, Vriens EM, Eikelboom BC, et al. Carotid endarterectomy with transcranial Doppler and electroencephalographic monitoring. A prospective study in 130 operations. Stroke 1993;24:665-669.

75. Spencer MP, Thomas GI, Moehring MA. Relationship between middle cerebral artery blood flow velocity and stump pressure during carotid endarterectomy. Stroke 1992; 23:1439-1445.

76. Kalra M, Al-Khaffaf H, Farrell A, et al. Comparison of measurement of stump pressure and transcranial measurement of flow velocity in the middle cerebral artery in carotid surgery. Ann Vasc Surg 1994;8:225-231.

77. Smith JL, Evans DH, Fan L, et al. Interpretation of embolic phenomena during carotid endarterectomy. Stroke 1995;26:2281-2284.

78. Hennerici MG. Can carotid endarterectomy be improved by neurovascular monitoring? Stroke 1993;24:637-638.

79. Halsey JH. Risks and benefits of shunting in carotid endarterectomy. Stroke 1992;23:1583-1587.

80. Arnold M, Sturzenegger M, Schaffler L, Seiler RW. Continuous intraoperative monitoring of middle cerebral artery blood flow velocities and electroencephalography during carotid endarterectomy. A comparison of the two methods to detect cerebral ischemia. Stroke 1997;28:1345-1350.

81. Gaunt ME, Naylor NR, Bell PRF. Preventing strokes associated with carotid endarterectomy: Detection of embolisation by transcranial Doppler monitoring. Eur J Endovasc Surg 1997;14:1-2.

82. Levi CR, O'Malley HM, Fell G, et al. Transcranial Doppler detected microembolism following carotid endarterectomy. High microembolic signal loads predicts postoperative cerebral ischaemia. Brain 1997; 120:621-629.

83. Magee TR, Davies AH, Baird RN, Horrocks M. A head box to protect transcranial Doppler transducers during carotid surgery. Eur J Vasc Surg 1992;6.

84. Spencer MP, Thomas GI, Nicholls SC, Sauvage LR. Detection of middle cerebral artery emboli during carotid endarterectomy using transcranial Doppler ultrasonography. Stroke 1990;21: 415-423.

85. Jansen C, Ramos LMP, van Heesewijk JPM, et al. Impact of microembolism and hemodynamic changes in the brain during carotid endarterectomy. Stroke 1994;25:992-997.

86. Gaunt ME, Martin PJ, Smith JL, et al. Clinical relevance of intraoperative embolization detected by transcranial Doppler sonography during carotid endarterectomy: a prospective study of 100 patients. Br J Surg 1994;81:1435-1439.

87. Ackerstaff RGA, Jansen C, Moll Fl, et al. The significance of microemboli detection by means of transcranial Doppler ultrasonography monitoring in carotid endarterectomy. J Vasc Surg 1995;21:963-969.

88. Smith JL, Evans DH, Fan L, et al. Interpretation of embolic phenomena during carotid endarterectomy. Stroke 1995;26:2281-2284.

89. Spencer MP. Transcranial Doppler monitoring and causes of stroke from carotid endarterectomy. Stroke 1997; 28:685-691.

90. Markus HS, Molloy J. Use of a decibel threshold in detecting Doppler embolic signals. Stroke 1997;28:692-695.

91. Powers AD, Smith RR. Hyperperfusion syndrome after carotid endarterectomy: a transcranial Doppler evaluation. Neurosurgery 1990;26:56-60.

92. Jorgensen LG, Schroeder TV. Defective cerebrovascular auto-regulation after carotid endarterectomy. Eur J Vasc Surg 1993;7:370-379.

93. Schaafsma A, Veen L, Vos JP. Three cases of hyperperfusion syndrome identified by daily transcranial Doppler investigation after carotid surgery. Eur J Vasc Surg 2002;23:17-22.

94. Lundar T, Lindegaard K-F, Froysaker T, et al. Cerebral perfusion during nonpulsatile cardiopulmonary bypass. Ann Thorac Surg 1985;40:144-150.

95. Lundar T. Transcranial Doppler in the study of cerebral perfusion during cardiopulmonary bypass. Chapter 11. In: Aaslid R (Ed), Transcranial Doppler Sonography_ New York, Springer-Verlag, 1986:164-172.

96. von Reutern G-M, Hetzel A, Birnbaum D, Schlosser V. Transcranial Doppler ultrasonography during cardiopulmonary bypass in patients with severe carotid stenosis or occlusion. Stroke 1988;19:674-680.

97. Padayachee TS, Parsons S, Theobold R, et al. The detection of microemboli in the middle cerebral artery during cardiopulmonary bypass: a transcranial Doppler ultrasound investigation using membrane and bubble oxygenators. Ann Throac Surg 1987;44:298-302.

98. Brass LM, Fayad PB. Chapter 17. Intraoperative monitoring with transcranial Doppler ultrasonography during cardiac surgery and interventions. In Babikian VL, Wechsler LR (eds): Transcranial Doppler Ultrasonography. St. Louis: Mosby, 1993:222-231.

99. Brackken SK, Russell D, Brucher R, et al. Cerebral microembolic signals during cardiopulmonary bypass surgery. Frequency, time of occurrence, and association with patient and surgical characteristics. Stroke 1997;28:1988-1992.

100. Barbut D, Hinton RB, Szatrowski TP, et al. Cerebral emboli detected during bypass surgery are associated with clamp removal. Stroke 1994;25:2398-2402.

101. Pusgsley W, Kinger L, Paschalis C, et al. The impact of microemboli during cardiopulmonary bypass on neuropsychological functioning. Stroke 1994;25:1393-1399.

102. Endoh H, Shimoji K. Changes in blood flow velocity in the middle cerebral artery during nonpulsatile hypothermic cardiopulmonary bypass. Stroke 1994;25:403-407.

103. Brillamn J, Davis D, Clark RE, et al. Increased middle cerebral arteryflow velocity during the initial phase of cardiopulmonary bypass may cause neurological dysfunction. J Neuroimaging 1995;5:135-141.

104. Barbut D, Yao FS ,Hager DN, et al. Comparison of transcranial Doppler ultrasonography and transesophageal echocardiography to monitor emboli during coronary artery bypass surgery. Stroke 1996;27:87-90.

105. Giller CA. Transcranial Doppler monitoring of cerebral blood flow velocity during craniotomy. Neurosurgery 1989;25:769-776.

106. Giller CA, Mathews D, Walker B, et al. Prediction of tolerance to carotid artery occlusion using transcranial Doppler ultrasound. J Neurosurg 1994;81:15-19.

107. Hurst RW, SchneeC, Raps EC, et al. Role of transcranial Doppler in neuroradiological treatment of intracranial vasospasm. Stroke 1993;24:299-303.

108. Schneweis S, Urbach H, Solymosi L, Ries F. Preoperative risk assessment for carotid occlusion by transcranial Doppler ultrasound. J Neurol Neurosurg Psychiatry. 1997;62:485-489.

109. Markus HS, Clifton A, Buckenham T, Brown MM. Carotid angioplasty. Detection of embolic signals during and after the procedure. Stroke 1994;25:2403-2406.

110. Giller CA, Prudy P, Giller A, et al. Elevated transcranial Doppler ultrasound velocities following therapeutic arterial dilation. Stroke 1995;26:123-127.

111. Giller CA, Steig P, Batjer HH, et al. Transcranial Doppler ultrasound as a guide to graded therapeutic occlusion of the carotid artery. Neurosurgery 1990;26:307-311.

112. Pfefferkorn T, Mayer T, Von Stuckrad-Barre S, et al. Hyperperfusion-induced intracerebral hemorrhage after carotid stenting documented by TCD. Neurology 2001;57:1933-1935.

113. Markus HS, Droste DW, Brown MM. Detection of asymptomatic cerebral embolic signals with Doppler ultrasound. Lancet 1994;343:1011-1012.

114. Siebler M, Kleinschmidt A, Sitzer M, et al. Cerebral microembolism in symptomatic and asymptomatic high-grade stenosis. Neurology 1994;44:615-618.

115. Siebler M, Nachtmann A, Sitzer M, et al. Cerebral microembolism and the risk of ischemia in asymptomatic high-grade stenosis. Stroke 1995;26:2184-2186.

116. Valton L, Larrue V, Arrue P, et al. Asymptomatic cerebral embolic signals in patients with carotid stenosis. Correlation with appearance of plaque ulceration on angiography. Stroke 1995;26:813-815.

117. Sitzer M, Muller W, Siebler M, et al. Plaque ulceration and lumen thrombus are the main source of cerebral microemboli in high-grade stenosis. Stroke 1995;26:1231-1233.

118. Lash S, Newell D, Mayber M, et al. Artery-to-artery cerebral emboli detection with transcranial Doppler: analysis of eight cases. J Stroke Cerebrovasc Dis 1993;3:15-22.

119. Grosset DG, Georgiadis D, Kelman AW, Less KR. Quantification of ultrasound emboli signals in patients with cardiac and carotid disease. Stroke 1993;24:1922-1924.

120. Tong DC, Bolger A, Albers GW. Incidence of transcranial Doppler-detected cerebral microemboli in patients referred for echocardiography. Stroke 1994;25:2138-2141.

121. Sliwka U, Job F-P, Wissuwa D, et al. Occurrence of transcranial Doppler high-intensity transient signals in patients with potential cardiac sources of embolism. A prospective study. Stroke 1995;26:2067-2070.

122. Siebler M, Stizer M, Rose G, et al. Silent cerebral embolism caused by neurologically symptomatic high-grade carotid stenosis. Brain 1993;116:1005-1015.

123. Georgiadis D, Kaps M, Siebler M, et al. Variability of Doppler microembolic signal counts in patients with prosthetic cardiac valves. Stroke 1995;26:439-443.

124. Muller HR, Lyrer P, Boccalini P. Doppler monitoring of middle cerebral artery emboli from carotid stenoses. J Neuroimaging 1995;5:71-75.

125. Nabavi DG, Georgiadis D, Mumme T, et al. Clinical relevance of intracranial microembolic signals in patients with left ventricular assist device. A prospective study. Stroke 1996;27:891-896.

126. Grosset DG, Georgiadis D, Abdullah I, et al. Doppler emboli signals vary according to stroke subtype. Stroke 1994;25:382-384.

127. Markus H. Transcranial Doppler detection of circulating cerebral emboli. A review. Stroke 1993; 24:1246-1250.

128. Forteza AM, Babikian VL, Hyde C, et al. Effect of time and cerebrovascular symptoms on the prevalence of microembolic signals in patients with cervical carotid stenosis. Stroke 1996;27:687-690.

129. Nabavi DG, Georgiadis D, Mumme T, et al. Detection of microembolic signals in patients with middle cerebral artery stenosis by means of a bigate probe. A pilot study. Stroke 1996; 27:1347-1349.

130. Eicke BM, Barth V, Kukowski B, et al. Cardiac microembolism: prevalence and clinical outcome. J Neurol Sci 1996;136:143-147.

131. Sliwka U, Lingnau A, Stohlmann W-D, et al. Prevalence and time course of microembolic signals in patients with acute stroke. A prospective study. Stroke 1997;28: 358-363.

132. Kaps M, Hansen J, Weither M, et al. Clinically silent microemboli in patients with artificial prosthetic aortic valves are predominantly gaseous and not solid. Stroke 1997;28:322-325.

133. Droste DW, Hagedorn G, Notzold A, et al. Bigated transcranial Doppler for the detection of clinically silent circulating emboli in normal persons and patients with prosthetic cardiac valves. Stroke 1997;28:588-592.

134. Koennecke H-C, Mast H, Trocio SS, et al. Microemboli in patients with vertebrobasilar ischemia. Association with vertebrobasilar and cardiac lesions. Stroke 1997;28:593-596.

135. Georgiadis D, Lindner A, Manz M, et al. Intracranial microembolic signals in 500 patients with potential cardiac or carotid embolic source and in normal controls. Stroke 1997;28:1203-1207.

136. Sliwa U, Klotzsch C, Popuscu O, et al. Do chronic middle cerebral artery stenoses represent an embolic focus? A multirange transcranial Doppler study. Stroke 1997;28:1324-1327.

137. Del Sette M, Angeli S, Stara I, et al. Microembolic signals with serial transcranial Doppler monitoring in acute focal ischemic deficit. A local phenomenon? Stroke 1997;28:1310-1313.

138. Babikian VL, Wijman CAC, Hyde C, et al. Cerebral microembolism and early recurrent cerebral or retinal ischemic events. Stroke 1997;28: 1314-1318.

139. Sliwka U, Georgiadis D. Clinical correlations of Doppler microembolic signals in patients with prosthetic cardiac valves. Analysis of 580 cases. Stroke 1998;29:140-143.

140. Babikian VL. Basic identification criteria of Doppler microembolic signals. Stroke 1995;26:1123.

141. Markus H, Bland JM, Rose G, et al. How good is intercenter agreement in the identification of embolic signals in carotid artery disease? Stroke 1996;27:1249-1252.

142. Markus HS, Ackerstaff R, Babikian V, et al. Intercenter agreement in reading Doppler embolic signals. A multicenter international study. Stroke 1997; 28:1307-1310.

143. Markus H. Importance of time-window overlap in the detection and analysis of embolic signals. Stroke 1995;26:2044-2047.

144. Droste DW, Markus HS, Nassiri D, Brown MM. The effect of velocity on the appearance of embolic signals studied in transcranial Doppler models. Stroke 1994;25:986-991.

145. Georgiadis D, Goeke J, Hill M, et al. A novel technique for identification of Doppler microembolic signals based on the coincidence method. In vitro and in vivo evaluation. Stroke 1996;27:683-686.

146. Bornstein NM, Krajewski A, Norris JW. Basilar artery blood flow in subclavian steal. Can J Neurol Sci 1988;15:417-419.

147. Hennerici M, Klemm C, Rautenberg W. The subclavian steal syndrome: A common vascular disorder with rare neurologic deficits. Neurol 1987;37(Suppl 1):316-317.

148. Klingeolhofer J, Conrad B, Benecke R, Frank B. Transcranial Doppler ultrasonography of carotid-basilar collateral circulation in subclavian steal. Stroke 1988; 19:1036-1042.

149. Thmassen L, Aarli JA. Subclavian steal phenomenon. Clinical and hemodynamic aspects. Acta Neurol Scand. 1994;90:241-244.

150. Berni A, Tromba L, Cavaiola S, et al. Classification of the subclavian steal syndrome with transcranial Doppler. J Cardiovasc Surg 1997;38:141-145.

151. Lindegaard K-F, Grolimund P, Aaslid R, Nornes H. Evaluation of cerebral AVM's using transcranial Doppler ultrasound. J Neurosurg 1986;65:335-344.

152. Petty GW, Massaro AR, Tatemichi TK, et al. Transcranial Doppler ultrasonographic changes after treatment for arteriovenous malformations. Stroke 1990;21:260-266.

153. Manchoa IF, DeSalles AAF, Foo TK, et al. Arteriovenous malformation hemodynamics: a transcranial Doppler study. Neurosurgery 1993;33:556-562.

154. Mast H, Mohr JP, Thompson JLP, et al. Transcranial Doppler ultrasonography in cerebral arteriovenous malformations. Stroke 1995;26:1024-1027.

155. Becker GM, Winkler J, Hoffmann E, Bogdahn U. Imaging of cerebral arterio-venous malformations by transcranial colour-coded real-time sonography. Neuroradiology 1990; 32:280-288.

156. Klotzsch C, Henkes H, Nahser HC, et al. Transcranial color-coded duplex sonography in cerebral arteriovenous malformations. Stroke 1995;26:2298-2301.

157. Adams RJ, Aaslid R, Gammal TE, et al. Detection of cerebral vasculopathy in sickle cell disease using transcranial Doppler ultrasonography and magnetic resonance imaging. Case report. Stroke 1988;19:518-520.

158. Adams R, McKie V, Nichols F, et al. The use of transcranial ultrasonography to predict stroke in sickle cell disease. N Engl J Med 1992;326:605-610.

159. Brass LM, Provhovnik I, Pavlakis SG, et al. Middle cerebral artery blood velocity and cerebral blood flow in sickle cell disease. Stroke 1991;22:27-30.

160. Siegel MJ, Luker GD, Glauser TA, DeBaun MR. Cerebral infarction in sickle cell disease: transcranial Doppler US versus neurologic examination. Radiology 197:191-194, 1995.

161. Venketasubramanian N, Prohovnik I, Hurlet A, et al. Middle cerebral artery velocity changes during transfusion in sickle cell anemia. Stroke 25:2153-2158, 1994.

162. Seibert JJ, Miller SF, Kirby RS, et al. Cerebrovascular disease in symptomatic and asymptomatic patients with sickle cell anemia: screening with duplex transcranial Doppler US-correlation with MR imaging and MR angiography. Neuroradiology 189:457-466, 1993.

163. Seibert JJ, Glasier CM, Kirby RS, et al. Transcranial Doppler, MRA, and MRI as a screening examination for cerebrovascular disease in patients with sickle cell anemia: an 8-year study. Pediatr Radiol28:138-142, 1998.

164. Adams R, McKie V, Hsu L, et al. Prevention of a first stroke by transfusions in children with sickle cell anemia and abnormal results on transcranial Doppler ultrasonography. N Engl J Med 339:5-11, 1998.

165. Jones AM, Seibert JJ, Nichols FT et al. Comparison of transcranial color Doppler imaging (TCDI) and transcranial Doppler (TCD) in children with sickle-cell anemia. Pediatr Radiol 2001;31:461-469.

166. Pegelow CH, Wang W, Granger S, et al. Silent infarcts in children with sickle cell anemia and abnormal cerebral artery velocity. Arch Neurol 58:2017-2021, 2001.

167. National Heart, Lung, and Blood Institute. Clinical alert issued for U.S. physicians: New treatment prevents stroke in children with sickle cell anemia.1997. September 18.

168. Neish AS, Blews DE, Simms CA et al. Screening for stroke in sickle cell anemia: comparison of transcranial Doppler imaging and nonimaging US techniques. Radiololgy 2002;222:709-714.

169. President's Commission.Guidelines for the determination of death. JAMA 246:2184-2186, 1981.

170. Ropper AH, Kehne SM, Wechsler L. Transcranial Doppler in brain death. Neurology 37:1733-1735, 1987.

171. Kirkham FJ, Levin SD, Padayachee TS, et al. Transcranial pulsed Doppler ultrasound findings in brainstem death. J Neurol, Neurosurg, and Psychiatry 50:1504-1513, 1987.

172. Hassler W, Steinmetz H, Gawlowski J. Transcranial Doppler ultrasonography in raised intracranial pressure and in intracranial circulatory arrest. J Neurosurg 68:745-751, 1988.

173. Powers AD, Graeber MC, Smith RR. Transcranial Doppler ultrasonography in the determination of brain death. Neurosurgery 24:884-889, 1989.

174. Newell DW, Grady MS, Sirotta P, Winn HR. Evaluation of brain death using transcranial Doppler. Neurosurgery 24:509-513, 1989.

175. Hassler W, Steinmetz H, Pirschel J. Transcranial Doppler study of intracranial circulatory arrest. J Neurosurg 71: 195-201, 1989.

176. Petty GW, Mohr JP, Pedley TA, et al. The role of transcranial Doppler in confirming brain death: sensitivity, specificity, and suggestions for performance and interpretation. Neurology 40:300-303,1990.

177. Lampl Y, Gilad R, Eschel Y et al. Diagnosing brain death using the transcranial Doppler with a transorbital approach. Arch Neurol 59:58-60, 2002.

178. Park CW, Sturzenegger M, Douville CM, et al. Autoregulatory response and CO2 reactivity of the basilar artery. Stroke 34:34-39, 2003.

Chapter 7
Case Examples

The following cases are examples of transcranial Doppler examinations from actual patients. Each report lists a representative mean velocity and a pulsatility index for each artery in the format: mean velocity/pulsatility index. For example in the first case; the right MCA has a mean velocity of 57 cm/sec and the pulsatility index is 0.7 (see circle below). A negative (-) value indicates blood flow away from the transducer (dotted circle below). In addition, questions follow each case report.

Case #1

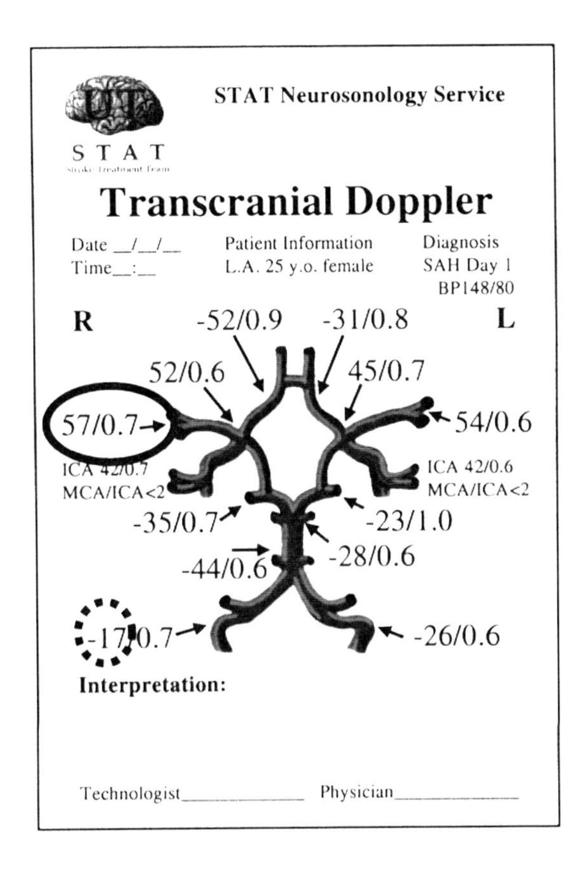

A 25 year old female with a Grade I subarachnoid hemorrhage (SAH) had a TCD examination performed on Day 1 following the onset of the patient's severe headache.

What is the interpretation? What is the normal range for the pulsatility index (P.I.) in adults?

Case #2

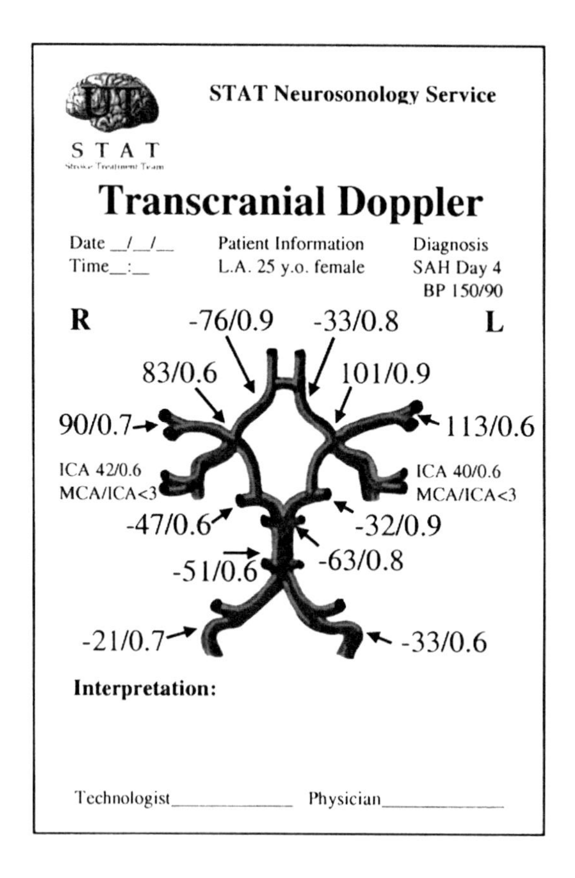
STAT Neurosonology Service

STAT

Stroke Treatment Team

Transcranial Doppler

Date __/__/__ Patient Information Diagnosis

Time__:__ L.A. 25 y.o. female SAH Day 4

BP 150/90

R **L**

-76/0.9 -33/0.8

83/0.6 101/0.9

90/0.7 113/0.6

ICA 42/0.6 ICA 40/0.6

MCA/ICA<3 MCA/ICA<3

-47/0.6 -32/0.9

-51/0.6 -63/0.8

-21/0.7 -33/0.6

Interpretation:

Technologist__________ Physician__________

A 25 year old female with a Grade I subarachnoid hemorrhage (SAH) had a TCD examination performed on Day 4. What is the interpretation?

What is the normal range for the mean velocity from the middle cerebral artery in adults?

Case #3

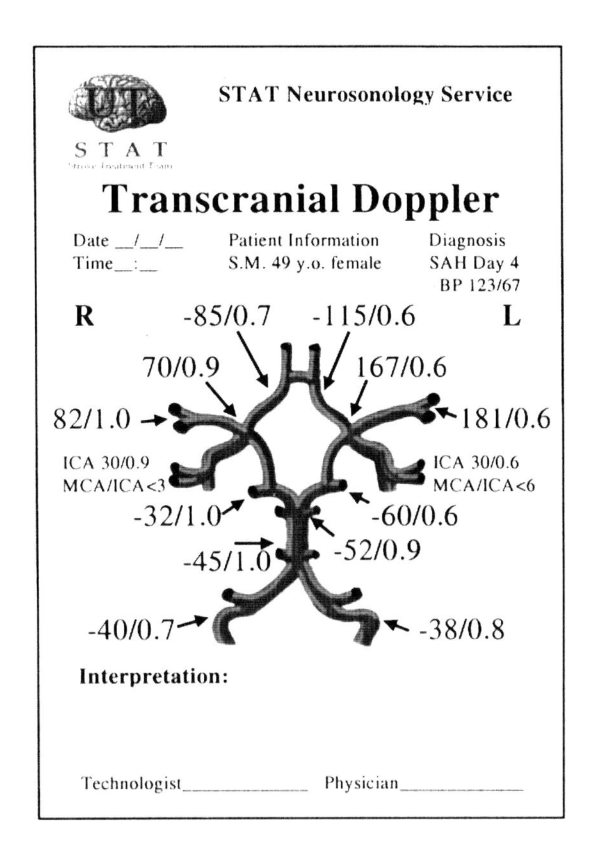
STAT Neurosonology Service

S T A T

Transcranial Doppler

Date __/__/__ Time__:__

Patient Information S.M. 49 y.o. female

Diagnosis SAH Day 4 BP 123/67

R L

-85/0.7 -115/0.6

70/0.9 167/0.6

82/1.0 181/0.6

ICA 30/0.9 MCA/ICA<3

ICA 30/0.6 MCA/ICA<6

-32/1.0 -60/0.6

-45/1.0 -52/0.9

-40/0.7 -38/0.8

Interpretation:

Technologist__________ Physician__________

A 49 year old female had a TCD examination performed on Day 4 following SAH after developing a severe headache. This patient had a Grade II SAH at onset.

What is the interpretation? What is the normal range for the Lindegaard ratio?

Case #4

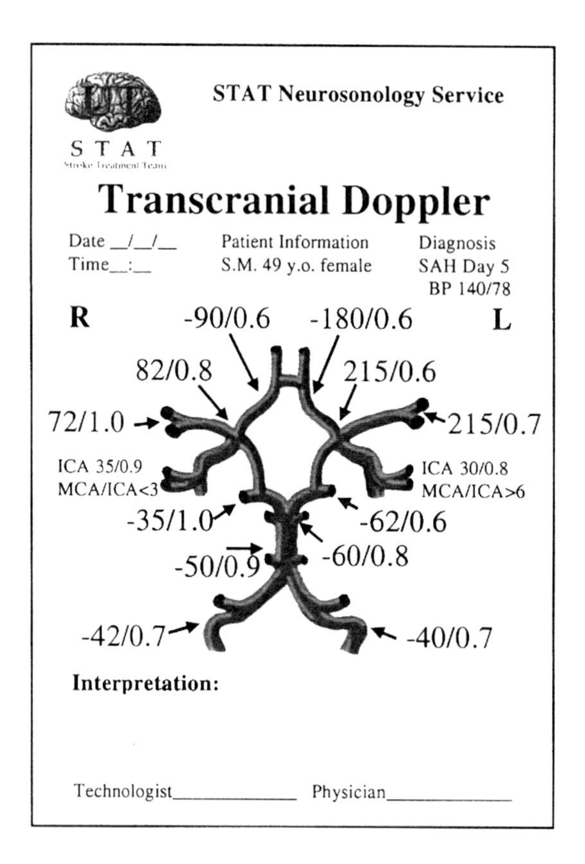

A 49 year old female had a TCD examination performed on Day 5 following SAH (same patient as in Case 3).

What is the interpretation? In this case, the increased velocities from the left ACA may indicate?

Case #5

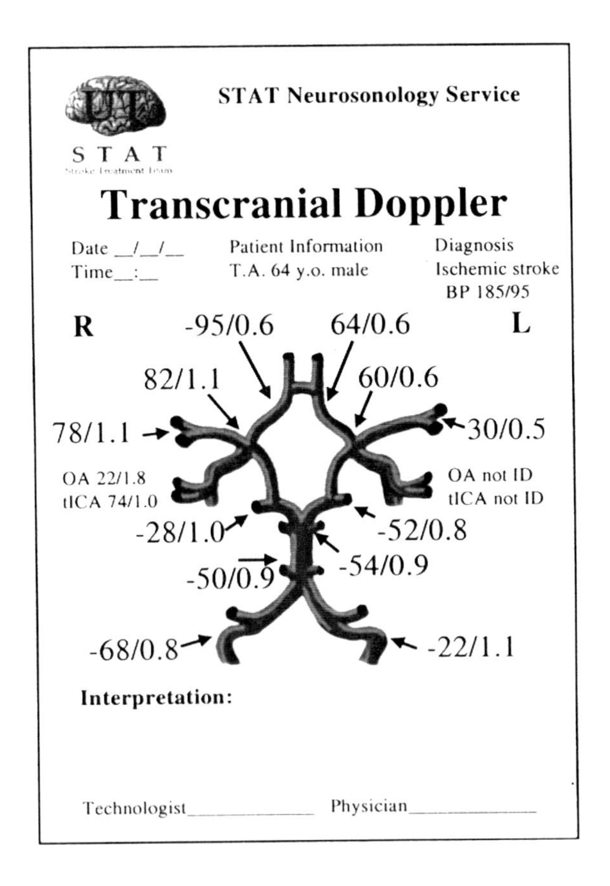
STAT Neurosonology Service

STAT

Transcranial Doppler

Date __/__/__ Patient Information Diagnosis
Time__:__ T.A. 64 y.o. male Ischemic stroke
BP 185/95

Interpretation:

Technologist____________ Physician____________

A 72 year old male who presented with an ischemic stroke had a TCD examination.

What is the interpretation?

Case #6

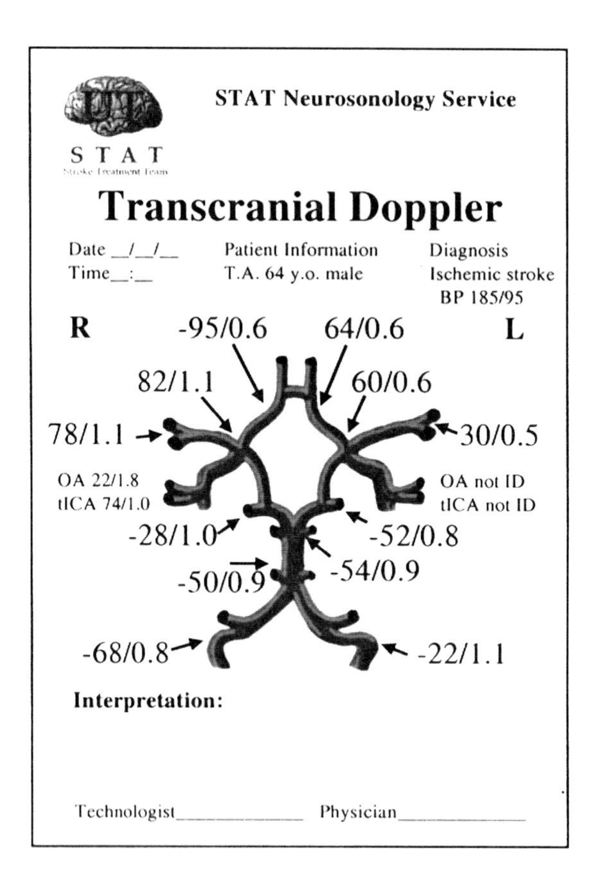

A 64 year old male who presented with an ischemic stroke had a TCD examination. No Doppler signal was obtained from the left ophthalmic artery or the terminal-ICA.

What is the interpretation? In this case, which collateral channels were identified?

Case #7

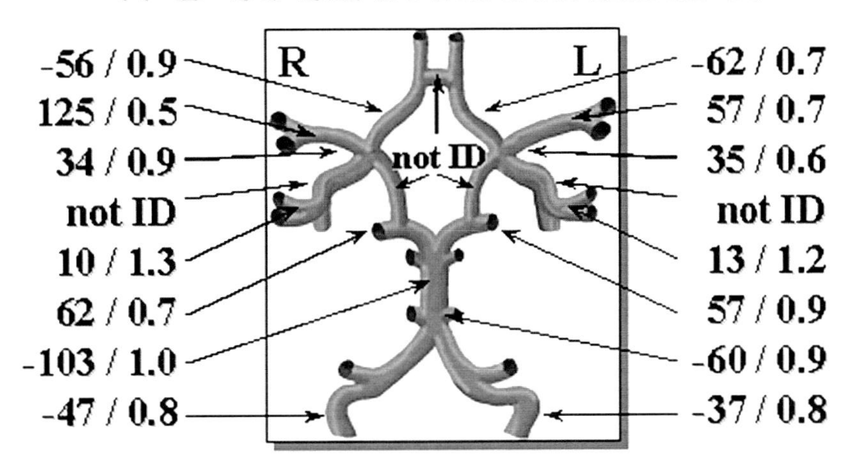

A 60 year old male presented with an ischemic stroke. During the TCD examination, no Doppler signal could be located via the transorbital window bilaterally. In addition, there was no evidence of collaterals.

What is the interpretation?

Case #8

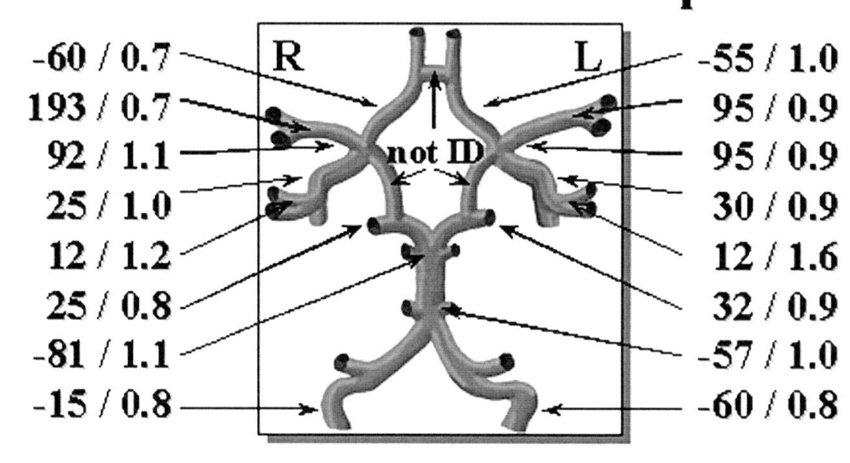

A 77 year old male s/p right carotid endarterectomy (1 week) presented with new mild right sided hemiparesis.

What is the interpretation?

Chapter 8
TCD Report Forms & Protocol

Considering the large quantity of hemodynamic information generated during a transcranial Doppler (TCD) or a transcranial color Doppler imaging examination, it is evident that the technologist/sonographer and interpreting physician must select from the data what is clinically important. Velocities (peak systolic, mean, end diastolic), pulsatility indices, velocity ratios, sample volume depths, direction of blood flow in relation to the transducer (away, toward, or bi-directional), response to CO2 inhalation can be recorded at numerous depth settings for each intracranial artery. This information should be consolidated in a clear and concise format.

This chapter describes: 1) how the TCD data may be recorded, 2) formats for TCD report forms, 3) what TCD information may be useful to the referring physician, and 4) a TCD examination protocol.

Data Collection

The information obtained during a transcranial Doppler and transcranial color Doppler imaging examination needs to be recorded and hard copy records may be obtained by different devices: 1) a printer, 2) photographs, 3) videotape, or 4) internal memory for later transfer to a computer. Whichever method is used to record the information during the examination, each Doppler spectral waveform should be clearly labeled for the right/left side and the intracranial artery. It is difficult, if not impossible, to remember the source of each Doppler spectral waveform after the examination is completed. A standard examination sequence avoids errors of omission and improves the ease with which the interpreter follows the examination. Following a TCD examination protocol is critical with multiple operators and interpreters.

Report Forms
Data Collection Form

Each institution should develop a standardized TCD data collection form. The information collected should include: the patient's name, hospital number, age, sex, race, medical and surgical history, presenting symptoms, indication for the examination, and space to record bilateral blood pressure, heart rate, the results of the extracranial carotid/vertebral studies, the postoperative day, and the date of the study. Intracranial pressure (ICP), $PaCO_2$, and hematocrit are also recorded when available. The values (depths, direction, mean velocity, P.I.,) from the spectral waveforms from each intracranial artery should be recorded. Using a well-designed data collection form simplifies the interpretation, and aids comparison of velocities from adjacent depths in the same artery and comparison of one side to the other at the same depth. A diagram of the Circle of Willis indicating direction of blood flow further assists with the rapid evaluation of collateral pathways.

Formal Report Form

Most physicians requesting a TCD examination do not know how to interpret the raw data generated during the examination. The data must be distilled so that the pertinent TCD data is reported in an organized and an understandable fashion. The final report must be clear and concise, so that the patient's

physician understands the clinically relevant information. Additionally, a formal report should have adequate patient identification (demographics), include an indication for the examination, and state any limitations of the examination.

Official TCD report forms vary and many list a single mean velocity and pulsatility index for each intracranial artery. Although values from only one depth setting may be listed for each intracranial artery, a thorough evaluation of each artery at several sample volume depths is required to confidently demonstrate significant findings (i.e. a focal increase in velocity).

Many formal TCD report forms have a diagram of the Circle of Willis so that blood flow direction can be marked with arrows. This allows for a visual display of the collateral pathways. Other report forms list the velocities, pulsatility indices, etc. in a column format allowing for quick comparison from artery to artery and from side to side. Although the formal report form will vary between institutions, the interpretation of the TCD data is obviously the most important part of the report. The interpretation conveys the clinically useful information to the referring physician.

TCD Interpretation

Interpreting the results of a TCD examination includes consideration of the various physiologic factors (i.e. age, hematocrit, etc.) that can influence intracranial arterial hemodynamics, the patient's neurologic signs and symptoms, and the results of the extracranial carotid/vertebral studies. Ideally, the TCD examination will provide information about intracranial arterial hemodynamics that will be helpful in patient management. Many referring physicians may not appreciate the importance of changes in the velocity or the pulsatility index of an intracranial arterial Doppler signal. Therefore, what will be useful to the referring physician is a description of the pertinent findings including the clinical implications. It is important for the interpreter to find a balance between relaying numbers and providing useful information to the referring physician. For example, if a significant focal increase in velocity and post stenotic turbulence is located in the middle cerebral artery, the interpretation should indicate that these findings suggest a stenosis of the MCA.

The interpretation of a TCD examination varies depending on the amount of hemodynamic information obtained from the patient. If an intracranial artery is not located or evaluated, it may be because of the technical limitations of the study, or an anatomic variant, and not inherent pathology, and the final report should reflect this limitation. With accurate accession, appropriate interpretation of the TCD data, and an appreciation of the limitations of the technique, physicians will become increasingly confident with the information the examination provides.

Summary

Since the complete TCD examination produces a large amount of hemodynamic information, the report form and subsequent interpretation must be clear and concise (Figures 8-1, 8-2). The most important points to remember when developing a TCD report form are to: 1) develop a format to efficiently record the essential hemodynamic information from each intracranial artery, and 2) provide a clinically relevant interpretation which is understood by the referring physicians.

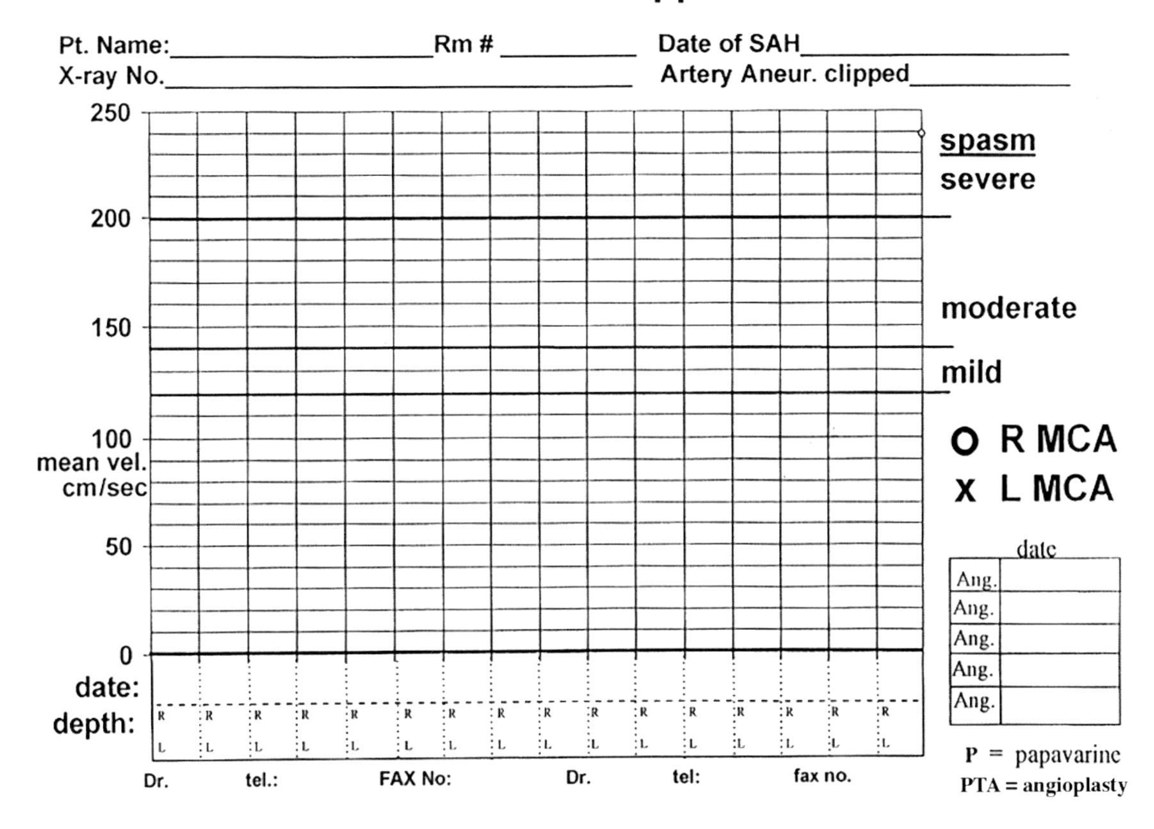

Figure 8-1. An example of a TCD report form used in monitoring vasospasm in MCAs post aneurysm clipping. (From Techniques in Noninvasive Vascular Diagnosis with permission of author).

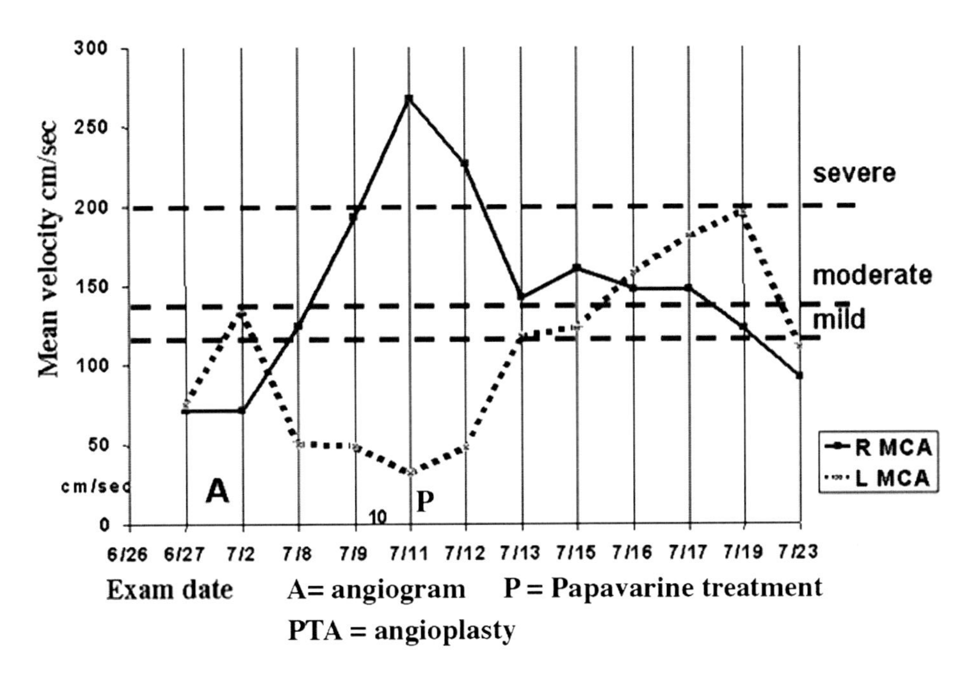

Figure 8-2. An example of a TCD vasospasm chart. (From Techniques in Noninvasive Vascular Diagnosis with permission of author).

TRANSCRANIAL DOPPLER STUDY

Patient Name ______________________________

Record # ____________________ Age ________ Sex ________

Date of Exam ____________ Physician ____________________

Presenting Condition ______________________________

____

Additional Exam Results ______________________________

____

____

HR ________ BP ________ ICP ________ $PaCO_2$ ________ Hct. ________ Post Op Day # ________

RIGHT PEAK-S / END-D	RIGHT MEAN	RIGHT PI	RIGHT DEPTH		LEFT PEAK-S / END-D	LEFT MEAN	LEFT PI	LEFT DEPTH
				OPHTHALMIC				
				SUPRACLINOID (SIPHON)				
				GENU (SIPHON)				
				PARASELLAR (SIPHON)				
				MCA 1				
				MCA 2				
				ACA				
				ACOA				
				ICA				
				PCA				
				PCOA				
				VA				
				BA				

– $\%CO_2$ (right) ________ – $\%CO_2$ (left) ________

Interpretation ______________________________

____

____

____

Figure 8-3. An example of a transcranial Doppler report form.

TCD Codes

The American Medical Association publishes the Current Procedural Terminology (CPT) Codebook. The following applies to TCD and TCDI and is from the 1999 CPT:

93886: Transcranial Doppler study of the intracranial arteries; complete study.

93888: Transcranial Doppler study of the intracranial arteries; limited study.

New for 2005:

93980: TCD vasoreactivity study

93892: TCD for emboli detection without bubble injection

93893: TCD for emboli detection WITH bubble injection.

TCD Examination Protocol

Purpose

The detection and monitoring of cerebrovascular disorders involving the intracranial arteries.

Equipment & Supplies

1) TCD non-imaging system (bidirectional pulsed Doppler) or a color Doppler imaging system.
2) Ultrasound transducers ranging from 1-2.5MHz.
3) Stereo Headphones.
4) Monitoring headset with appropriate transducer.
5) Examination table or stretcher.
6) Hardcopy devices: video-recorder, printer, computer, etc.
7) Ultrasound gel, transducer disinfectant.
8) Clean towels.
9) TCD report forms.

Indications

The indications for the TCD examination will vary depending on clinical considerations. Some of the indications for the TCD examination include the following:

1) Suspected intracranial disease (stenosis, occlusion, aneurysm, AVMs).
2) Stroke or TIA.
3) Screening children with sickle cell disease.
4) Monitoring,
   (vasospasm in subarachnoid hemorrhage, intraoperative, emboli detection, evolution of cerebral circulatory arrest, fibrinolytic therapy, neuroradiology procedures)

Contraindications

1) Transorbital window: The evaluation using this TCD approach usually should not be performed if the patient has a history (less than one year) of recent eye surgery. Consult the patient's ophthalmologist.

Procedure

1) Explain the TCD examination to the patient and answer any questions.
2) Obtain the results of the patient's extracranial arterial evaluation.
3) Obtain a brief cerebrovascular history and record on the TCD report form. Include the patient's medical (hypertension, diabetes, obesity, hyperlipidemia, smoking, etc.) and surgical history (cardiac, carotid endarterectomy, etc.), presenting signs and symptoms, hematocrit, ICP, and a summary of previous TCD test results.

Equipment/Patient setup

1) Input patient demographics and the date into the ultrasound system and on report forms.
2) Choose the proper ultrasound transducer and the manufacturers presets for the TCD examination.
3) Find a comfortable position for the patient. The best results will be obtained with the patient lying in the supine position with their head resting on a small pillow. The patient should be placed on their side and with their head bowed slightly toward their chest for evaluation via the suboccipital approach.
4) The TCD operator should find a comfortable position that allows access to the patient and the equipment.

The Examination

1) The transcranial Doppler examination of the intracranial arteries is performed via four ultrasound windows (transtemporal, transorbital, suboccipital, and submandibular).
2) Complete bilateral examinations should be performed in all cases, unless technically impossible. If a limited examination is performed, an explanation for the limitation is documented.
3) A zero degree angle is assumed during the examination.
4) The power output of the equipment is reduced for evaluation via the transorbital window. A mechanical index of 0.28 or less (10% power on some equipment) must be used for the evaluation via the orbital approach. The ALARA principle applies.
5) At each depth setting, record the best quality Doppler signal possible. Adjustment in transducer angle and position and the various instrument controls (gain, PRF, etc.) may be necessary to obtain the best quality Doppler signal. Each intracranial artery is evaluated along its entire length. Hardcopy of the Doppler spectral waveform from each intracranial artery must be obtained.
6) The intracranial arteries identified from each TCD window are listed below.

Window	Artery
Transtemporal	Middle Cerebral Anterior Cerebral Anterior Communicating Terminal Internal Carotid Posterior Cerebral Posterior Communicating
Transorbital	Ophthalmic Internal Carotid (siphon)
Suboccipital	Vertebral Basilar
Submandibular	Internal Carotid

7) In adults, the depth of each intracranial artery and the direction of blood flow relative to the transducer are listed below:

Artery	Depth (mm)	Direction
MCA	30-67	Toward
ACA (A1)	60-80	Away
t-ICA	60-67	Toward
PCA (P1)	55-80	Toward
Ophthalmic	40-60	Toward
Carotid siphon	60-80	Toward, Away, Bidirectional
Vertebral	40-85	Away
Basilar	>80	Away
ICA (submandibular)	35-70	Away

8) In adults, the mean velocity for each intracranial artery is listed below:

Artery	Mean velocity (cm/sec)
MCA	62 ±12
ACA	50 ±11
t-ICA	39 ± 9
PCA	39 ±10
Ophthalmic	21 ± 5
Carotid siphon	47 ±14
Vertebral	38 ±10
Basilar	41 ±10
ICA (submandibular)	37 ± 9

9) The ACoA and PCoA are only located when these vessels are being used as a collateral pathway.
10) Wipe the ultrasound gel off the patient with a clean towel.
11) Wipe the excess ultrasound gel off the TCD transducer and use a disinfectant.

Interpretation

1) Each intracranial artery is examined along its length (multiple sample volume depths) and the mean velocity and pulsatility index (P.I.) are recorded on the data collection form.

2) A complete TCD examination is performed bilaterally. If an intracranial window or artery is not located, reasons for the technical limitation should be reported.

3) Interpretation of the TCD/TCDI examination is based on the spectral Doppler waveforms. Characteristics of the Doppler waveform that aid in the interpretation are: a) the depth of the sample volume, b) direction of blood flow relative to the transducer, c) the mean velocity, and d) the pulsatility index (P.I.).

4) The normal depth ranges, direction of blood flow relative to the transducer, and the mean velocity for adults are listed above (examination section). The normal P.I. ranges from 0.5 – 1.1.

5) The difference in mean velocity between sides is normally less than 30%.

6) Intracranial arterial velocities decrease with increasing age.

7) Increases in intracranial arterial velocities (global) will be present if the hematocrit is less than 30%.

8) Normal intracranial arterial velocity hierarchy is MCA>ACA>PCA>BA>VA.

9) In children, the intracranial arterial depth ranges and mean velocities will vary with age.

10) Intracranial stenosis: a focal increase in velocity with post-stenotic turbulence. An intracranial stenosis is suspected if the velocity is greater than 80 cm/sec in the anterior circulation and 70 cm/sec in the posterior circulation.

11) Collateral patterns:
a) ACoA: increase in ACA velocity on the contralateral side of the high-grade stenosis/occlusion, reverse flow direction in the ipsilateral ACA, and a turbulent Doppler signal at midline. b) PCoA:Increased velocity. c) ECA-ICA: reverse flow direction and achange from increased pulsatility to a low resistance signal in the ophthalmic artery.

12) Vasospasm:

-Mild: 100-119 cm/sec,
MCA/ICA ratio of 3

-Moderate: 120-199 cm/sec,
MCA/ICA ratio >3 and < 6.

-Severe: greater than 200 cm/sec,
MCA/ICA ratio ≥ 6

13) Children with sickle cell disease: Mean velocities in the MCA/t-ICA of <170 cm/sec is normal, 170-199 cm/sec is conditional, and ≥ 200 cm/sec is abnormal.

14) Reporting of TCD results: A preliminary report is written in the progress notes of the patient's chart and the referring physician is called if clinically indicated. A final, official interpretation of the TCD study should be completed within 24 hours.

15) Correlation with intracranial arteriography/ MRA is routinely performed on an ongoing basis. Dissemination of information to medical and technical personnel of the laboratory is performed on a routine basis.

16) The TCD examination protocol listed above is the basic standard procedure that provides the information necessary for a complete intracranial arterial evaluation. Special clinical indications may require a modification of the technique to obtain satisfactory and clinically relevant information for a patient. Modification of the standard technique should be recorded and reported.

Comprehensive Examination

1) When performing TCD examinations, the best results will be obtained using a _______ transducer.

   a) 10 MHz
   b) 10 KHz
   c) 5 KHz
   d) 5 MHz
   e) 2 KHz
   f) 2 MHz

2) List the four TCD ultrasound "windows".

____

____

____

____

3) The large terminal branch of the internal carotid artery is the __________ artery.

   a) Anterior cerebral
   b) Middle cerebral
   c) Posterior cerebral
   d) Ophthalmic
   e) Posterior communicating

4) The foramen magnum is a large opening in the _________ bone.

   a) Temporal
   b) Occipital
   c) Ethmoid
   d) Tibia
   e) Frontal

5) The union of the two vertebral arteries form the __________ artery.

   a) Basilar
   b) Posterior cerebral
   c) Posterior communicating
   d) Posterior inferior cerebellar
   e) Anterior inferior cerebellar

6) In the traditional TCD spectral Doppler waveform, blood flow away from the transducer is displayed ________ the zero baseline.

a) Above
b) Below
c) Equal to

7) A _______ degree angle is assumed when performing TCD examinations.

a) 0
b) 25
c) 45
d) 60
e) 100

8) Intracranial arterial velocities ________ with increasing age.

a) Increase
b) Decrease
c) Expand
d) Do not change

9) Hyperventilation causes a(n) _______ in the MCA velocity and a(n) _______ in the pulsatility index.

a) Increase
b) Decrease
c) No change

10) The anterior cerebral artery is normally located from the __________ approach. The depth of the artery is usually ______ mm, and blood flow is normally _______ the transducer.

a) Transtemporal
b) Suboccipital
c) Transorbital
d) Submandibular
e) 30-50
f) 60-80
g) 80-100
h) 100-120
i) Toward
j) Away from
k) Bi-directional to

11) A _______ Doppler transducer is used fo TCD examinations.

a) Pulsed
b) Continuous wave
c) Alternating
d) Mechanical

12) A low hematocrit (<30%) is associated with _______ intracranial arterial velocities.

a) Increased
b) Decreased
c) No change in the

13) The two A1 segments of the anterior cerebral artery (ACA) are joined by the ________.

a) A2 segment of the right ACA
b) Anterior communicating artery
c) A2 segment of the left ACA
d) Recurrent artery of Heubner

14) The acoustical intensity should be ________ to evaluate the carotid siphon using the transorbital approach.

a) Increased
b) Decreased
c) Set to normal

15) Using the suboccipital approach, blood flow is normally _____ the transducer in the vertebrobasilar system.

a) Toward
b) Away from
c) Bi-directional to

16) Name three intracranial collateral pathways that can be identified during a TCD examination.

____

____

____

17) Most TCD users report _______ velocities during TCD examinations.

a) Peak systolic
b) Mean
c) End diastolic
d) Pulsatility

18) When performing a transcranial color Doppler imaging examination, via the transtemporal approach, the intracranial bony landmarks used to locate the terminal portion of the internal carotid artery are the ________ and the _______.

a) Occipital bone
b) Petrous ridge of the temporal bone
c) Sphenoid wing
d) Ethmoid bone
e) Frontal bone

19) The _______ artery wraps around the cerebral peduncles.

a) Middle cerebral
b) Anterior cerebral
c) Anterior communicating
d) Posterior cerebral
e) Posterior communicating

20) The ability to penetrate the temporal bone by ultrasound is influenced by the age, sex, and race of the patient. It is more difficult to penetrate the temporal bone in _______, _______, and _______ patients.

a) Smaller
b) Younger
c) Older
d) Males
e) Females
f) African American
g) Caucasian

21) An ACA/MCA ratio greater than _______ is indicative of a pathologic situation present in the anterior cerebral artery.

a) 0.5
b) 1.2
c) 2.0
d) 3.0
e) 6.0

22) When the ophthalmic artery is being used as a collateral pathway from the external carotid artery to the internal carotid artery, blood flow will be ________ the transducer.

a) Toward
b) Away from
c) Bi-directional to

23) To eliminate aliasing from a Doppler spectral waveform, the operator should _______ the pulse repetition frequency.

a) Increase
b) Decrease
c) Not adjust

24) Why is maintaining patient comfort important during a TCD examination?

a) Maximizes ultrasound penetration
b) Avoids reflection
c) Minimizes aliasing
d) Avoids hypocapnia or hypercapnia

25) As intracranial pressure increases, pulsatility _____ and mean velocity ________.

a) Decreases
b) Increases
c) Does not change
d) Expands

26) The operator sets the color gain ______ to detect intracranial arterial blood flow during TCDI examinations.

a) Low
b) High

27) Side-to-side differences that occur during a TCD examination should be considered within normal limits if they are less than _____ percent.

a) 25
b) 50
c) 75
d) 100

28) When evaluating patients for vasospasm following subarachnoid hemorrhage, an MCA/ICA (cervical) ratio of greater than ______ indicates severe vasospasm.

a) 1.0
b) 2.0
c) 3.0
d) 4.0
e) 5.0
f) 6.0

29) The to-and-fro Doppler signal is characteristic of _____ peripheral vascular resistance.

a) Increased
b) Decreased
c) No change in

30) When evaluating arteriovenous malformations, the "feeding" arteries demonstrate ________ in velocity and _______ in the pulsatility index.

a) An increase
b) A decrease
c) No change

31) After evaluating the MCA, the color PRF may need to be _____ to evaluate the PCA. Why?

a) Increased
b) Decreased

32) The hemodynamic change associated with a significant intracranial stenosis is a(n) _______ velocity at the narrowed segment.

a) Increased
b) Decreased

33) The interpretation of the transcranial color Doppler imaging examination is made from the ______.

a) Gray scale image
b) Color Doppler display
c) Doppler spectral waveforms
d) Color bar

34) Middle cerebral artery velocities (cm/sec) of _____ correlate with severe vasospasm.

a) 40-70
b) 60-80
c) > 100
d) > 120
e) > 180
f) > 200

35) When evaluating an area of stenosis, the pulse repetition frequency will usually need to be _____.

a) Increased
b) Decreased
c) Not adjusted

36) List three technical modifications the operator can perform when trying to locate a TCD window.

____

____

____

37) List three sources of error in the diagnosis of an intracranial stenosis or occlusion.

____

____

____

38) The pulsatility index (P.I.) of the middle cerebral artery is normally in the range of:

a) 0-0.6
b) 0.5-1.1
c) 1.6-2.6
d) 2.0-3.0
e) 3.0-4.0

39) When evaluating the intracranial arteries, the TCD operator should sample the Doppler signal at _____ mm steps.

a) 2-5
b) 5-10
c) 10-15
d) 15-20

40) During a transcranial Doppler examination, the patient lowers their head toward their chest for the evaluation of the suboccipital approach. Why?

a) Patient balance
b) Prevent motion artifact
c) Enlarge the ultrasound window
d) Prevent Doppler aliasing

41) A bi-directional Doppler signal found at the midline via the transtemporal window represents blood flow in the _______ artery bilaterally.

a) Middle cerebral
b) Anterior cerebral
c) Posterior communicating
d) Vertebral

42) When evaluating a patient for vasospasm, which of the following is a possible reason for a false negative TCD examination?

d) Decreased velocities are not detected by current equipment
e) The middle cerebral artery is routinely displaced in these patients
c) TCD bedside examinations are not reliable
d) Vasospasm is occurring in the distal branches

43) List five clinical applications for using TCD.

____

____

____

____

____

44) List two limitations and two advantages of using transcranial color Doppler imaging.

____

____

____

____

45) How can the operator differentiate between an intracranial arterial stenosis and vasospasm?

46) A "classic" Circle of Willis is found in approximately _____ percent of the cases.

a) 100
b) 75
c) 50
d) 25

47) Why is the diagnosis of arterial occlusion limited to the MCA when performing a TCD examination?

48) A Doppler spectral waveform is obtained via the transtemporal window from a normal volunteer. The signal demonstrates blood flow toward the transducer. How would you determine if the Doppler signal is from the MCA or the PCA?

49) Why is the use of headphones recommended when performing TCD examinations?

50) List the window, depth, and direction of blood flow relative to the transducer for the following intracranial arteries:

MCA, ACA, PCA, Ophthalmic, Vertebral, Basilar

Answers
Cases and Comprehensive Examination

Cases

Case#	Interpretation
1	No evidence of vasospasm. (Normal range for P.I. is 0.5 – 1.1.)
2	Hyperemia throughout the intracranial arterial system. (Normal MCA mean velocities: 62 ± 12 cm/sec.)
3	Moderate left MCA (M1) vasospasm. (Normal Lindegaard ratio: <3)
4	Severe left MCA (M1) vasospasm. (ACA vasospasm, t-ICA bifurcation vasospasm, compensatory velocity increase)
5	Right MCA (M1) stenosis.
6	Terminal-ICA occlusion on the left side. There is evidence of right-to-left cross-filling via the Anterior Communicating Artery.
7	Right MCA and mid Basilar artery stenoses.
8	Right MCA, Left MCA, and Basilar artery stenoses. No evidence of collateral channels detected.

Comprehensive Examination

1) f
2) Transtemporal, Transorbital, Suboccipital, Submandibular
3) b
4) b
5) a
6) b
7) a
8) b
9) b, a
10) a, f, j
11) a
12) a
13) b
14) b
15) b
16) hemisphere – hemisphere (via anterior communicating artery); anterior – posterior (via posterior communicating artery); and external carotid artery – internal carotid artery (via ophthalmic artery)
17) b
18) b, c
19) d
20) c, e, f
21) b
22) b
23) a
24) d
25) b, a
26) b
27) a
28) f
29) a
30) a, b
31) b, PCA has lower velocities than the MCA
32) a

Comprehensive Examination (cont.)

33) c
34) f
35) a
36) 1. Move ultrasound transducer slowly along the skin.
    2. Angle the ultrasound transducer.
    3. Change the depth of the sample volume.
37) 1. Misinterpreting collateral channels or vasospasm as stenoses (vasospasm usually involves several arteries and the velocities change with time).
    2. The technical limitations of evaluating distal branch disease (stenosis or occlusion).
    3. The misinterpretation of a tortuous or displaced MCA (by hematoma or tumor) diagnosed as an occlusion.
    4. Anatomic variability (location, asymmetry, tortuousity), especially in the vertebrobasilar system.
    5. Technical difficulty in the evaluation of the distal basilar artery.
    6. Poor quality arteriography leading to inaccurate correlation of the TCD results.
38) b
39) a
40) c
41) b
42) d
43) Diagnosis of intracranial vascular disease, Monitoring vasospasm in subarachnoid hemorrhage, Screening of children with sickle cell disease, Assessment of intracranial collateral pathways, Evaluation of the hemodynamic effects of extracranial occlusive disease on intracranial blood flow, Detection of cerebral emboli, Monitoring evolution of cerebral circulatory arrest, Documentation of subclavian steal, Evaluation of the vertebrobasilar system, Detection of feeders of arteriovenous malformations (AVMs), Monitoring anticoagulation regimens or thrombolytic therapy, Monitoring during neuroradiologic interventions, Testing of functional reserve.
44) Limitations: operator experience, improper instrument controls, patient movement Advantages: provides anatomic guidance, documents location of the Doppler spectral waveform, visualization of M2 branches, vertebral artery confluence, collateral pathways, etc.

45) The intracranial arterial velocities associated with vasospasm will change with time and usually involve several arteries.

46) d

47) Inadequate transtemporal windows, anatomic variability

48) "Trace" the anatomic route of the artery. MCA is expected at 30-67mm and the PCA at 55-75mm.

49) Very high velocities are difficult to hear and the headphones block out extraneous background noise.

50) MCA (transtemporal window, 30-67 mm, toward); ACA (transtemporal window, 60-80 mm, away); PCA (transtemporal window, 55-75 mm, toward); Ophthalmic (transorbital window, 40-60 mm, toward); Vertebral (suboccipital window, 40-85 mm, away); Basilar (suboccipital window, >80 mm, away)

Index

A

acoustic output 67
age 1, 2, 32, 60, 81, 84, 85, 87, 88, 91, 101, 102,
ALARA 27, 140
aliasing 26, 52, 53, 56
aneurysms 64, 71, 93, 94, 99, 98, 106, 137, 139
angle 29, 30, 31, 32, 33, 34, 36, 37, 41
anterior cerebral artery (ACA) 9, 13, 15, 17, 18, 34, 35, 36, 40, 42 63, 92, 95, 96, 117
anterior communicating artery (ACoA) 14, 15, 17, 36, 37, 64, 95, 96, 99
aortic arch 11, 19
arteriovenous malformation 4, 71, 88, 91, 110, 155
artifacts 67, 100, 104, 107
attenuation 25, 32, 60, 100
autoregulatory response 97

B

basilar artery 10, 14, 16, 17, 21, 41, 42, 63, 65, 66, 67, 69, 71, 94, 97, 101, 108, 109
brain activity. 87
brain death 53, 113, 114
bruits 52, 84, 93

C

carbon dioxide 82, 85, 97, 98, 116
carotid duplex imaging 1, 2, 3, 4, 38, 81, 107
carotid siphon 39, 40, 42, 60, 67, 68, 92
cerebellar 37, 41, 67
cerebral emboli 105
circle of Willis 9, 14, 15, 16, 17, 18, 50, 59, 62, 63, 71, 87, 135, 136, 151
CO2 reactivity 98
collateral pathways 38, 69, 80, 91, 94, 135, 136
color box 50, 53, 65
color map 50
common carotid artery 2, 3, 4, 11, 12, 13, 17, 38
common carotid artery compression 4
compression 4, 8, 38, 42, 50, 106

D

data collection 85, 135, 141
Doppler gain 26, 92, 104, 107
duplex imaging 2, 3, 50, 53, 68, 81
dynamic range 50

E

ensemble length 53
equipment 25, 26, 28, 29, 33, 35, 38, 42, 43, 45, 49, 54, 55, 67, 69, 71, 83, 84, 98, 99, 103, 114, 139, 140
examination sites 58
external carotid artery 3, 11, 12, 13, 17, 19

F

fever 85
focal zone 50, 65
frame rate 50, 53, 65

G

gain 25, 26, 28, 49, 51, 52, 53, 56, 62, 65, 67, 92, 104, 107
gender 84
genu 13, 14, 15, 39, 40, 67, 68
gray scale image 49, 50, 53, 62, 65

H

hematocrit 2, 84, 85, 87, 88, 91, 100, 101, 135, 136, 139, 141
HITS 104, 108
hyperventilation 85, 86, 144
hypoglycemia 85

I

innominate artery 108
internal carotid artery (ICA) 2, 3, 4, 9, 10, 11, 12, 13, 14, 15, 17, 18, 27, 34, 36, 38, 39, 40, 42, 43, 54, 62, 68, 95, 97, 98, 103, 111, 116
intima-media thickness 3
intracranial arterial stenosis 91

L

limitations 43, 44, 49, 68, 69, 83, 87 88, 94, 108

M

M-mode 1,5,27,47
MCA/ICA ratio 100, 141
mechanical index 56, 67, 140
middle cerebral artery 9, 13, 14, 15, 18, 26, 28, 33, 34, 35, 36, 37, 38 44, 52, 54, 62, 70, 72, 77, 91, 92, 97, 99, 100, 102, 103, 111, 112, 113, 136

N

Nyquist limit 26, 52, 53, 56

O

OA 39, 68, 95
occipital bone 60
operator 79, 80, 86, 92, 94, 97, 103
ophthalmic artery (OA) 10, 12, 13, 14, 38, 39, 60, 67, 68, 95, 96, 130, 141
output 26, 56, 107, 112

P

parasellar 13, 39, 40, 67, 68
peduncles 59, 63
persistence 53, 65
petrous 59, 62
posterior cerebral artery 9, 14, 16, 17, 18, 21,37, 38, 42, 63, 64, 72, 92, 99
posterior communicating artery (PCoA) 13, 14, 17, 20, 37, 63, 64, 95, 96, 141
power 1, 25, 27, 32, 112, 140
power Doppler 53, 64, 70, 72, 94
PRF (see pulse repition frequency)
priority 53
pulsatility index 25, 28, 39, 54, 83, 88, 136, 1 41
pulse repetition frequency (PRF) 26, 50, 52, 55, 56, 71
pulsed Doppler 52, 53, 139

R

reactivity 85, 97, 98
resistance index 83, 84

S

sample volume depth 25, 26, 34, 35, 37, 41, 54, 55, 59, 69, 72, 79, 101
sample volume size 25, 43, 55, 79, 84, 102, 112
sex 32, 60, 84, 89, 135
sickle cell 4, 44, 71, 91, 111,139, 142
spatial peak 56, 67
spectral broadening 26, 55, 84
sphenoid bone 59, 62
stroke 1, 3, 44, 70, 71, 74, 97, 98, 101, 104, 105, 106, 108, 111
subarachnoid hemorrhage 4, 42, 82, 91, 98, 101, 110, 115, 125, 126, 13 9, 155
subclavian steal 4, 91, 108, 109, 124
submandibular window 42, 68
suboccipital window 40, 41, 65
supraclinoid 12, 13, 20, 39, 40, 68
supraorbital artery 10, 14

T

t-ICA 34, 35, 37
TCD Interpretation 136
TCD monitoring 97, 101, 102, 103, 104, 105, 108
temporal bone 31, 58, 59, 60, 62, 69, 84, 113
terminal ICA bifurcation 33, 36, 37, 38, 61, 92
thrombolytic therapy 5
transducer angle 39, 61, 79, 140
transducer orientation 67
transorbital window 27, 38, 56, 60, 67, 131, 139, 140
transtemporal window 32, 33, 34, 36, 40, 45, 47, 80, 92, 99, 100, 103, 104, 112, 114

U

ultrasound windows 30, 31,58, 69, 140

V

vasospasm 4, 44, 69, 82, 88, 89, 91, 94, 98, 99, 100, 101, 110, 114, 137, 148, 149, 150, 1 51, 153, 155
veins 18, 21, 22, 23, 51, 71, 110
velocity Ratios 82, 100, 135
vertebral arteries 2, 10, 11, 16, 17, 40, 41, 42, 65, 66, 67, 101, 108, 109
vertebrobasilar 4, 42, 60, 65, 66, 91, 92, 94, 109

W

wall filter 51, 56, 71

Z

zygomatic arch 33, 60, 61